PROCEDURES IN
INFANTS *and*
CHILDREN

PROCEDURES IN
INFANTS *and*
CHILDREN

▼

Michele C. Walsh-Sukys, M.D.
Associate Professor of Pediatrics
Division of Neonatology
Rainbow Babies and Childrens Hospital
Case Western Reserve University
Cleveland, Ohio

Steven E. Krug, M.D.
Associate Professor of Pediatrics
Northwestern University
Head, Pediatric Emergency Medicine
Children's Memorial Medical Center
Chicago, Illinois

Nancy A. Burgard, M.A., Medical Illustrator
Cleveland, Ohio

W.B. SAUNDERS COMPANY
A Division of Harcourt Brace & Company
Philadelphia • London • Toronto • Montreal • Sydney • Tokyo

W.B. SAUNDERS COMPANY
A Division of Harcourt Brace & Company

The Curtis Center
Independence Square West
Philadelphia, Pennsylvania 19106

Library of Congress Cataloging-in-Publication Data

Walsh-Sukys, Michele C.

Procedures in infants and children / Michele C. Walsh-Sukys, Steven E. Krug.

p.   cm.

ISBN 0–7216–3789–2

1. Children—Surgery.   2. Therapeutics, Surgical.   3. Infants—Surgery.
I. Krug, Steven E.   II. Title. [DNLM: 1. Surgery, Operative—in
infancy & childhood.   2. Therapeutics—in infancy & childhood.
WO 925 W228p 1997]

RD137.W35   1997   617.9′8—dc21

DNLM/DLC   96-48725

PROCEDURES IN INFANTS AND CHILDREN   ISBN 0-7216-3789-2

Printed in the United States of America.

Last digit is the print number: 9   8   7   6   5   4   3   2   1

NOTICE

Pediatrics is an ever-changing field. Standard safety precautions must be followed, but as new research and clinical experience broaden our knowledge, changes in treatment and drug therapy become necessary or appropriate. Readers are advised to check the product information currently provided by the manufacturer of each drug to be administered to verify the recommended dose, the method and duration of administration, and contraindications. It is the responsibility of the treating physician relying on experience and knowledge of the patient to determine dosages and the best treatment for the patient. Neither the Publisher nor the editor assumes any responsibility for any injury and/or damage to persons or property.

The Publisher

CONTRIBUTORS

David E. Bank, M.D.
Assistant Professor of Pediatrics, Columbia College of Physicians and Surgeons; Director, Pediatric Emergency Services, Roosevelt Hospital, New York, New York

Mary Barkey, M.S., C.C.L.S.
Child Life Specialist, Department of Family and Child Life, Rainbow Babies and Childrens Hospital, Cleveland, Ohio

Patty Batchelder, R.N., M.S.N., C.C.R.N.
Nurse Practitioner, Pediatric Neurosurgery, Columbia Presbyterian, St. Luke's Medical Center, Denver, Colorado

Jim R. Harley, M.D.
Assistant Clinical Professor of Pediatrics, University of California, San Diego; Attending Emergency Physician, Children's Hospital of San Diego, San Diego, California

Cynthia Hoecker, M.D.
Assistant Clinical Professor of Pediatrics, University of California, San Diego; Attending Emergency Physician, Children's Hospital of San Diego, San Diego, California

Brenda R. Hook, M.D.
Assistant Professor of Pediatrics, University of Texas Health Science Center, Houston, Texas

John T. Kanegaye, M.D.
Assistant Clinical Professor of Pediatrics, University of California, San Diego; Attending Emergency Physician, Children's Hospital of San Diego, San Diego, California

Sally Lambert, Ph.D., R.N.
Clinical Nurse Specialist, Rainbow Babies and Childrens Hospital, Cleveland, Ohio

Timothy Mapstone, M.D.
Associate Professor of Surgery, Department of Pediatric Neurosurgery, University of Alabama, The Children's Hospital of Alabama, Birmingham at Birmingham, Alabama

Celeste M. Marx, Pharm. D.
Assistant Professor of Pediatrics, Rainbow Babies and Childrens Hospital, Case Western Reserve University, Cleveland, Ohio

Ian McCaslin, M.D.
Assistant Clinical Professor, Department of Pediatrics, University of California, San Diego; Attending Emergency Physician, Children's Hospital of San Diego, San Diego, California

Sally L. Reynolds
Associate Director, Emergency Department, Children's Memorial Hospital, Chicago, Illinois

Barbara Stephens, R.N., M.S.N.
Department of Pediatric Nursing, Rainbow Babies and Childrens Hospital, Cleveland, Ohio

Anita H. Weiss, M.D.
Assistant Professor of Pediatrics, Division of Pharmacology and Critical Care, Case Western Reserve University, Rainbow Babies and Childrens Hospital, Cleveland, Ohio

PREFACE

"The art is long, and life is short"
Hippocrates

"See one, do one, teach one"
Anonymous

Conventional textbooks in medicine focus nearly exclusively on the cognitive aspects of practice. Students and residents generally learn procedures from one another in the *"see one, do one, teach one"* school of medicine. We have prepared this text to instruct students, residents, and practitioners in the art and science of pediatric procedures in a more systematic way. Because much of this learning requires visual information, the text relies heavily on illustration. We are deeply indebted to the talented artist Nancy Burgard for the superb illustrations.

We have combined our professional expertise with that of our contributors from across the country to produce a text that will serve the pediatrician well in his or her practice from the newborn to the adolescent with trauma. It is our hope that by seeking input from contributors across the country we have achieved a broad perspective rather than a parochial one.

During the preparation of the text, we have been reminded of the countless lessons we have received from our talented mentors, colleagues, and students. We have also reflected on the extreme demands and the indescribable rewards experienced by all who have the privilege of helping sick children recover and thrive. Our patients are our ultimate teachers, our joy, our strength.

MWS
SEK

ACKNOWLEDGMENTS

It has been said that writing a book takes twice the effort and four times as long as one planned; that is certainly the case with this one. We thank:

- Our families, Sean, Ryan, Lori, Alex, and Lindsey, for their grace and patience.
- Our colleagues, for their thoughtful critiques.
- Our residents and students of all kinds: pediatric residents and medical students, nurse practitioners, critical care nurse transporters, and paramedics for challenging us to expand our teaching skills.
- Our ever-patient and encouraging editor, Lisette Bralow.
- And most importantly our patients: the children who inspire us with their courage and fortitude.

MWS
SEK

CONTENTS

SECTION 1

PREPARATION

CHAPTER 1

Anita H. Weiss

INFORMED CONSENT

Informed consent is of fundamental importance to the practice of modern medicine, so much so that it is considered the ethical and legal cornerstone of the contemporary physician-patient relationship.[1] In contrast to the traditional relationship between physicians and patients that was characterized by unilateral choices of physicians who "knew what was best" for their patients, the current physician-patient relationship is defined by mutual respect and by participation of both physician and patient in the process of decision making.[1,2]

Because most pediatric patients have neither the capacity nor the legal power to consent to medical treatment on their own, the application of informed consent is more complicated in pediatric clinical medicine and in research involving children. However, the concept of informed consent has also become essential to the ethical and legal practice of pediatrics by defining the relationships among pediatrician, parent, and patient.[3]

WHAT IS INFORMED CONSENT?

Informed consent is predicated on the moral principle of respect for persons, called *respect for autonomy.*[4-6] Its primary function is to facilitate and safeguard the autonomous choice of legally competent patients.[6] Rather than defining informed consent per se, it is better to conceptualize it as a process that fulfills all the following criteria as set forth by Faden, Beauchamp, and King:[4]

1. "A patient or subject must agree to an intervention based on an understanding of (usually disclosed) relevant information.
2. Consent must not be controlled by influences that would engineer the outcome.
3. The consent must involve the intentional giving of permission for an intervention."

The informed consent process as described earlier necessitates meaningful communication of relevant information between the physician and patient.[7] Such discussion should focus on the "course medical care should take."[1] It is inappropriate to think of informed consent only as a legal formality or a superficial recitation of inconsequential or obscure medical facts.[1] True informed consent also cannot be guaranteed by a patient's signature on a written consent form.[1]

Rather, informed consent should be considered a process of responsible decision making by legally competent patients (or their surrogates) that is both supported and assisted by the physician. Its purpose is to promote patients' fundamental right to know about their health, to know about the risks and benefits of appropriate treatment or diagnostic options, and to choose among appropriate options or even to refuse them.[4, 8] As such, the informed consent process has profound significance for patients as well as physicians.

THE LEGAL, MEDICAL, AND MORAL BACKGROUND OF INFORMED CONSENT

The legal background of informed consent came from the English common law of the mid-1700s, which prohibited nonconsensual touching, considered a culpable battery under the law.[2, 9]

> *Under the battery theory a defendant is held liable for any intended (i.e., not careless or accidental) action that results in physical contact for which the plaintiff has given no permission.*[7]

No exception was made for medical treatment except in the case of emergencies.[2] Therefore, any physician who performs a nonemergent invasive procedure without a patient's permission could be liable for battery, even though the procedure was performed competently and even though most people probably would have agreed to the procedure.[7] Thus, the early legal formation of informed consent was primarily concerned with unauthorized procedures and the avoidance of liability for battery rather than with the nature of patients' understanding or the authenticity of their consent.[2, 4, 7]

Later legal standards became concerned with the physician's obligation to disclose information to the patient.[16] Two different legal standards emerged regarding the nature and amount of information physicians should disclose. These are the professional practice standard and the reasonable person standard.[7]

The *professional practice standard* defines the amount of information that must be disclosed to a patient by the established norm of the medical professional community.[5, 7] In other words, it is the information that a fictional "reasonable physician" would disclose to an average patient about the medical risks and the benefits of and the alternatives to the procedure or treatment in question. The *reasonable person standard* (sometimes called the *lay standard* or *material risk approach*), however, is more patient-oriented. It is concerned with the information a fictional "reasonable patient" would want and need to know about the medical risks and benefits of and the alternatives to the procedure or treatment in order to formulate a responsible decision about whether or not to undergo the procedure or treatment.[5, 7]

In contrast to its lengthy history in the law, informed consent is a relatively new concept in medicine: the term did not even appear in the medical literature until 1957 and was not discussed as the concept is currently considered until as late as 1972.[7] However, over the next 20 years informed consent became so important that it is now considered a fundamental legal and bioethical requirement for research and clinical medicine. Some authors equate these events in medicine to the movement toward greater individual freedom and self-determination that took place in our society during the 1960s and 1970s.[2]

Substantial differences also exist between the legal and ethical perspectives of informed consent. The legal viewpoint emphasizes the obligation of physicians to inform patients and obtain their consent before all nonemergent procedures and medical treatments.[4] The ethical viewpoint, however, goes beyond physician disclosure of information. In ethics, the goal of informed consent is to *encourage the patient's autonomous choice*[4, 6] and to *improve the patient's understanding* about the proposed procedure or medical treatment.[7] To accomplish these goals, physicians must do more than merely disclose information. They must provide complete and understandable explanations, encourage meaningful discussion, explain reasonable alternatives, and present a recommended course of action to *help the patient make a responsible decision.*[2]

In this context, the sum and substance of informed consent is respect for individual autonomy. This is accomplished by respecting patients' ability to define their own goals and values and by respecting their ability to make choices consistent with those goals and values.[2] According to Beauchamp and Childress:[6]

> *Any definition that makes disclosure the chief condition (of informed consent) incorporates dubious assumptions about medical authority, about physician responsibility, or about legal theories of liability, all of which delineate an* obligation *to make disclosures rather than a* meaning *of informed consent. The meaning of informed consent ... is better analyzed in terms of autonomous authorization.*

MODELS OF PROXY CONSENT

The concept of informed consent just discussed applies to patients who are legally competent and thus empowered by law to give an informed consent. When a patient is legally incapable of informed consent, referred to as being *legally incompetent,* a designated person may make medical decisions for the incompetent patient. This is called *proxy consent* or *surrogate decision making.*

Whenever a surrogate makes a medical decision for an incompetent patient, the ethical principles of *beneficence* (helping the patient) and *nonmaleficence* (avoidance of harming the patient) are generally used to guide the surrogate's decision.[6] To help accomplish the difficult task of making medical decisions for incompetent persons, two different but related proxy decision-making standards have been used: the substituted judgment doctrine and the best interests standard.

The *substituted judgment doctrine* requires the proxy decision maker to make the decision. Although it takes some imagination, this model attempts to take into account the actual circumstances of the incompetent person's life to arrive at the decision the incompetent person would have made if he or she were competent. This model of surrogate decision making, therefore, uses respect for the incompetent person's autonomy and privacy as primary ethical guidelines for the medical decision.[6]

The *best interests standard* takes a different approach to surrogate decision making. It uses the objective standard of the ordinary person[10] and concepts such as risk, harm, and benefit to guide surrogate decisions for incompetent patients.[6] In contrast to the substituted judgment doctrine, the best interests model relies on the ethical principles of beneficence and nonmaleficence; it requires the surrogate decision maker to choose the option that is in the best interests of the incompetent person. The best interests model is less interested in trying to figure out what the incompetent patient would have decided if he or she were competent and is, therefore, less concerned with the autonomy of the incompetent person.

CONSENT IN PEDIATRICS: PARENTAL PROXY CONSENT

When making health-care decisions for children, it is important to remember that *competence,* the empowerment to give informed consent, is a legal definition based on common law and statute. By law, a child is presumed incompetent until the legal age of majority. This means that the traditional concept of informed consent cannot be applied to neonatal and most pediatric patients because these patients are "below the age of legal majority" and they do not (with some exceptions that will be discussed later in this section) possess the full capacity or the legal empowerment to give an informed consent.

Therefore, in pediatrics, a surrogate decision maker must make medical decisions for the minor child. Usually the surrogate is the child's parent, although other individuals or the courts can act as surrogates in specific circumstances. Consequently, informed consent in pediatrics has traditionally represented the process of obtaining permission for the medical procedure or treatment from the child's parent or guardian on behalf of the minor child. This process is called *parental proxy consent.* (Some contemporary commentators believe it is more precise to call this process *informed parental permission.*[11])

There is longstanding history and tradition to support parents as the most appropriate decision makers for minor children. Historically, children were considered the chattel (or property) of their parents.[12] Today, it is recognized that parents must make decisions on their children's behalf in order to fulfill their responsibilities to their children.[13] Practical considerations also support parents as the most appropriate decision makers for their minor children. For example, parents live intimately with the consequences of medical decisions affecting their children, they are responsible for the well-being of their children, and, as they are close relatives to their children, they fulfill next-of-kin criteria as surrogate decision makers.[13]

There are also important moral reasons to support parents as decision makers for their minor children. According to Capron:[10]

> *Parents achieve their position as substitutes because they are likely best to know their child's existing views and the value preferences of the family unit, which typically play the leading role in molding the child's future views.*

This viewpoint recognizes the interrelated nature of the interests, values, and preferences of the child, parent, and family. It attempts to apply the ethical value of respect for autonomy to young children and their families, even though young children are considered legally "incapable" of being autonomous and require their parents to make decisions on their behalf.

Despite this long history and tradition, the pragmatic considerations and moral reasoning that support parents as the most appropriate surrogate decision makers for minor children, several problems with the concept of parental proxy consent have been identified. The first problem is that parental authority over children is not absolute; there are several legal limits to parental authority. For example, parents must provide their children with an education (although they are given wide discretion about how to do so), there are laws about childhood vaccinations, parents must obey child abuse and neglect statutes, and the judicial system has interceded when parents have refused standard medical therapy for children with life-threatening illnesses.[13]

Another difficulty with the concept of parental proxy consent concerns the actual efficacy of the traditional models of proxy decision making (the best interests standard and substituted judgment doctrine). When considering the best interests standard for the proxy decisions of parents, it is important to recognize that parents have interests separate from those of their children, which may conflict with, or impair, the parents' ability to make reasonable choices for their child.[14, 15]

The substituted judgment doctrine has also been considered inadequate for patients who have never been competent to express a preference about treatment, such as young children.[6] It is debatable whether an adult can ever really "know the child's mind," as the doctrine requires.[15] For these reasons it is controversial whether either or both the best interests standard and the substituted judgment doctrine can completely ensure that adequate medical decisions will be made for minors.

For decisions that affect the health and well-being of neonatal and pediatric patients, one should also ask: What is the role of the health-care team? Although the parent is the primary decision maker for the child, the health-care team plays an important role as independent advocate for the life, health, and well-being of the child. Furthermore, pediatricians' principal ethical obligation is to promote the best interests of their minor patients.[16, 17]

This obligation requires the health-care team to work closely with parents so the best decisions can be made for children. This may involve explanation and discussion, care conferences, support from nursing, social service or child life personnel, the clergy, or bioethics consultation. When parents' refusal of standard medical treatment seriously jeopardizes the life or health of a child, this refusal does not relieve the health-care team of responsibility or negate their primary obligation to the child.[17] In these cases, intervention from appropriate social agencies or from the courts may be necessary to protect the health or life of the child.[11, 12]

CHILD ASSENT

Owing to the aforementioned concerns and the recognition of children as developing individuals with growing capacity for making decisions, some authors have advocated for greater participation of children in the health-care decision-making process.[3, 11, 14, 17, 18] This process is called *child assent.*

The main goal of child assent is to involve children in their medical care to the extent of their individual capacity.[4, 11] It attempts to maximize the child's involvement in their medical care and to allow some aspects of medical treatment to be placed within the child's control.[3]

The philosophy of child assent recognizes children's varying decision-making capacity, depending on their age, maturity, intellect, and the nature of the decision.[3, 14] As such, the process of child assent takes into account the developmental capacities and maturity of the child while continuing to respect the unique role of the parent and family in the decision-making process.[3, 13, 15]

Child assent is *not* a substitute for parental permission for medical treatment of minor children. *The parents or guardian remain the primary decision makers* in these matters, especially for young children. However, this approach to medical decision making has several humanistic, therapeutic, and pragmatic advantages over traditional parental proxy consent. For this process to succeed, excellent communication must exist among the child, parent, and physician.

Child assent recognizes the need of children to be aware of their medical condition and to participate in the decision-making process, even though the child may not be legally competent to give consent.[14, 17] The process attempts to include the child in communication about health-care decisions in a manner that is consistent with the child's age and level of maturity; children should be given the information necessary to acquire an age-appropriate understanding of their medical condition and the proposed procedure or medical treatment.[11] When appropriate, the process of child assent may also include solicitation of the willingness of the child to participate in the procedure or medical treatment.[11, 17]

Proponents of child assent believe attainment of full capacity for informed consent (legal competency) is a developmental task of childhood,[3, 17] and that the pediatrician's role includes an obligation to help children prepare for the future as a competent adult decision maker in the health-care arena. Child assent allows children to learn to participate in age-appropriate communication about health-care and medical decisions with the support of parents and medical staff.[3]

EMANCIPATED MINORS, MATURE MINOR DOCTRINE, MINOR TREATMENT STATUTES, AND EMERGENCY MEDICAL TREATMENT OF MINORS

There are several exceptions to the general rule of parental consent in pediatrics. These are as follows: the emancipated minor, the minor treatment statutes, the mature minor rule, and emergency treatment of minor children.

Emancipated minors are children who are "not subject to parental control or regulation."[12] Although the exact legal definition varies, emancipation usually involves minors who are not living at home, are not dependent financially on their parents, and whose parents have relinquished parental authority.[11] Emancipated minors can legally give informed consent for medical treatment without parental permission.

In some states adolescents who are mature and capable of understanding the risks, purpose, and nature of a medical intervention may authorize treatment in some situations: this is called the *mature minor doctrine.*[19] Although the actual age to which the doctrine applies varies, according to Sigman and O'Connor, "under this doctrine, minors who are able to understand the nature and consequences of the medical treatment offered are considered mature enough to consent to or refuse the treatment."[19] Before consent can be accepted from an adolescent under this doctrine the physician is obligated to balance the maturity of the adolescent against the nature of the medical decision. Consequently, this doctrine generally applies only to medical interventions that involve little risk and are intended directly to benefit the adolescent. In regard to major and high-risk medical interventions, court orders have still been required before consent could be accepted from an adolescent.[19]

Some states also have laws that allow minors to consent for treatment of specific conditions such as drug and alcohol abuse, mental illness, pregnancy, contraception, and sexually transmitted diseases. These laws are called *minor treatment statutes.* They are intended to promote the medical care and treatment of minors who might otherwise not seek medical attention because of anxiety, fear, or embarrassment.[19] Health-care professionals who care for adolescents should learn the laws regarding mature minors and minor treatment statutes in the states where they practice.

Physicians may also give medical care to minor patients in emergency situations, when attempts to contact parents were unsuccessful or could not be accomplished in time. According to Holder, in these instances emergencies are defined as "anything requiring relatively urgent attention or causing pain or fear"[12] although the exact legal definition may vary.[19]

CONCLUSION

A patient who has been "informed" has received and understands the information needed to make a responsible decision about the proposed medical treatment or procedure. The patient has given consent when he or she freely agrees, without coercion from others, to proceed with the procedure or treatment.

Informed consent in pediatrics is more complicated because most pediatric patients (with some exceptions) cannot consent on their own for medical procedures and treatment. In these circumstances, parents or guardians are asked to give proxy consent or informed permission on behalf of the minor. Parents and medical staff should help the child understand what will occur during the procedure or treatment and solicit the child's assent or cooperation when appropriate. This approach to medical care allows "informed parental consent" to occur while helping the child achieve a better understanding of his or her illness, what will happen during the procedure or treatment and the need for the procedure or treatment. For this process to succeed, open and honest communication must exist among the physician or medical staff, parent, and child.

Whenever pediatric patients are empowered to give informed consent, such as emancipated minors or competent pediatric patients who are above the age of legal majority, their consent or refusal of medical procedures and treatment should be honored.

Respect for the process of informed consent denotes respect for patients and their families: respect for patients' personal values and life goals and their freedom to live according to those values and goals within the limits of our society.

Acknowledgments

I would like to thank Rebecca S. Dresser, JD, and Jeffrey L. Blumer, PhD, MD, for their kind support and helpful guidance with the preparation of this manuscript.

References

1. Jonsen AR, Siegler M, Winslade WJ. Clinical ethics: A practical approach to ethical decisions in clinical medicine. New York, Macmillan, 1986.
2. President's Commission for the Study of Ethical Problems in Medicine and Biomedical and Behavioral Research. Making health care decisions: A report on the ethical and legal implications of informed consent in the patient-practitioner relationship. Washington, DC, US Government Printing Office, 1982.
3. King NMP, Cross AW. Children as decision makers: Guidelines for pediatricians. J Pediatr 115:10–16, 1989.
4. Faden RR, Beauchamp TL, King NMP. A history and theory of informed consent. New York, Oxford University Press, 1986.
5. Sprung CL, Winick BJ. Informed consent in theory and practice: Legal and medical perspectives on the informed consent doctrine and a proposed reconceptualization. Crit Care Med 17:1346–1354, 1989.
6. Beauchamp TL, Childress JF. Principles of biomedical ethics. New York, Oxford University Press, 1989.
7. Beauchamp TL. Informed consent. In Veatch RM (ed). *Medical Ethics.* Boston, Jones and Bartlett, 1989.
8. American Hospital Association. Statement on a patient's bill of rights. Hospitals 47:41, 1973.
9. Radetsky M. The doctrine of informed consent. In Nussbaum E (ed). *Pediatric Intensive Care.* Armonk, NY, Futura Publishing, 1989.
10. Capron AM. The authority of others to decide about biomedical interventions with incompetents. In Gaylin W, Macklin R (eds). *Who Speaks for the Child: The Problems of Proxy Consent.* New York, Plenum Press, 1982.
11. Bartholome WG. A new understanding of consent in pediatric practice: consent, parental permission, and child assent. Pediatr Ann 18:262-265, 1989.
12. Holder AR. Disclosure and consent problems in pediatrics. Law Med Health Care 16:219-228, 1988.
13. Forman EN, Ladd RE. Ethical dilemmas in pediatrics: A case study approach. New York, Springer-Verlag, 1991.

14. Leikin S. A proposal concerning decisions to forgo life-sustaining treatment for young people. J Pediatr 115:17–22, 1989.
15. Fost NC. Children and biomedicine. In Reich WT (ed). *Encyclopedia of Bioethics.* New York, The Free Press, 1978.
16. American Academy of Pediatrics Committee on Bioethics. Treatment of critically ill newborns. Pediatrics 72:565–566,1983.
17. American Academy of Pediatrics Committee on Bioethics. Informed consent, parental permission, and assent in pediatric practice. Pediatrics 95:314–317, 1995.
18. Leikin SL. Minors' assent or dissent to medical treatment. J Pediatr 102:128–135, 1983.
19. Sigman GS, O'Connor C. Exploration for physicians of the mature minor doctrine. J Pediatr 119:520–525, 1991.

CHAPTER 2

Sally Lambert
Barbara Stephens
Mary Barkey
Michele Walsh-Sukys

NONPHARMACOLOGIC PAIN RELIEF

DO CHILDREN FEEL PAIN?

Children are brought to the hospital for relief of pain and suffering. Unfortunately, their experiences in the hospital setting frequently result in more pain and distress. For a variety of reasons pain, especially in infants and children, is frequently undertreated, even in children's hospitals, which should be expert in their care. Some common misinformation may contribute to this undertreatment. Many caretakers incorrectly assume that children have immature neurologic systems that are not capable of responding to pain. Research has now conclusively documented that even the most premature infant senses and mounts a biologic response to pain. Another myth that interferes with adequate pain relief is that children metabolize analgesics differently from adults, and in fact may be harmed more by analgesics than they are helped. By 1 month of age, children demonstrate pharmacokinetics that are identical to those of adults. Younger infants can be safely treated using analgesics, as with all other drugs, by using appropriate dosages (see Chapter 3).

Another obstacle to adequate relief of children's pain is the difficulty of assessing pain in children, particularly in those who are preverbal. Children may not have the language to make caregivers aware of their pain, and even those who do may not express their feelings because they are unaware that relief is possible or because they are worried that they will get a "shot" if they acknowledge their pain. Three different approaches to pain assessment in children are currently used: (1) physiologic assessments that take into account various vital sign measures such as heart rate and blood pressure, which may correlate with pain; (2) behavioral observations that score groups of behaviors; and (3) visual scales in which the child is asked to rate his or her pain by pointing to pictures representing different degrees of discomfort (i.e., smiling faces through grimacing faces). If children say they are in pain, we should believe them.

Research in the area of children's pain is now receiving increasing attention in the literature. Pain is also beginning to be addressed in the medical and nursing curriculum. Recent attention of the lay press to the topic and the publication of clinical practice guidelines by the Agency for Health Care Policy and Research have each contributed to heightened awareness among professionals.

Thus, children do feel pain, which can be adequately treated with pharmacologic agents and supplemented with nonpharmacologic approaches that are easily incorporated into practice. It is incumbent on children's caregivers to become knowledgeable regarding these techniques and to ensure their use.

As every adult knows, pain is not just a neurosensory experience but is modified by one's state and perceptions. Similarly children's perception of pain may be influenced by age, cognitive development, previous experiences with painful procedures, parental support, and the physical environment in which the interaction occurs. Children exhibit a developmental progression in their understanding of pain that parallels the sophistication of their cognitive development (Table 2-1). Therefore, different ages will require different supportive approaches. Most infants and children will benefit from the support of their parents' physical presence during the procedure. Adolescents should also be given the option to have their parents accompany them. If the parent is not available, another familiar caretaker may partially fulfill this supportive role. Some physicians are uncomfortable allowing parents to be present during procedures. We have found, however, that a well-coached parent is a significant ally rather than an impediment to the procedure, and usually saves time and enhances cooperation. In our institution, a large pediatric teaching hospital, we follow a "three strikes and you are out" rule. Any person performing a procedure, regardless of their level of training or expertise, is allowed no more than three attempts before a more experienced individual is recruited. (Of course, in many situations, no attempt is made when the degree of difficulty is assessed by the operator to be beyond his or her technical expertise.) This rule has become incorporated in our institutional culture and is followed by even the most senior attending physician. In this manner, trauma to the child is minimized and parents are reassured that their child's best interests are served.

STEPS TO MINIMIZE ACUTE PAIN ASSOCIATED WITH PROCEDURES

1. Provide a comfortable nonthreatening environment located away from the child's hospital room and the play room. Children's security is threatened during hospitalization. This threat can be ameliorated by creating areas that are "safe havens" where children know that no painful procedures will be performed, and they can relax in safety. Whenever possible, give the child some control over the procedure by providing choices such as "Do you want to sit on this side of the table or on that side?"

Table 2–1. **DEVELOPMENTAL SEQUENCE OF UNDERSTANDING OF PAIN**

Age	Understanding
0–3 mo	No apparent understanding of pain; memory for pain likely but not conclusively demonstrated; responses perceptually dominated
3–6 mo	Pain response of infancy supplemented by toddler anger response
6–18 mo	Developing fear of painful situations; words common for pain including "ouchie," "booboo"; localization of some pain
Up to 6 yr	Prelogical thinking characterized by concrete thinking, egocentrism, and transductive logic
7–10 yr	Concrete operational thinking characterized by child being able to distinguish self from environment; use of behavioral coping strategies
11+ yr	Formal logical thinking, characterized by abstract thinking and introspection; increased use of mental or cognitive coping strategies

From McGrath PA, Craig KD. Developmental and psychological factors in children's pain. Pediatr Clin North Am 36:823–836, 1989.

2. Prepare the parent and child for the procedure by providing an explanation in lay terms of the procedure that is appropriate to the child's age. Be sure to explain why the procedure is necessary. Honesty is indeed the best policy: if it will hurt, say so. Emphasize the ways in which you will help the child deal with the pain. Prepare the child for sights, sounds, and physical sensations he or she will experience.

3. Behavioral strategies can help children work through anticipated or previously experienced pain. In general, children as well as adults are less fearful when they know what to anticipate. Therefore, role playing or demonstrating the procedure on a doll is effective with a young child, whereas watching a video tape that models the procedure may be more effective with an older child or adolescent.

4. The child's age often determines the most effective behavioral strategy (Table 2-2). Neonates and infants can be comforted with a pacifier and with swaddling. Recently oral sucrose administration prior to a procedure has been found to have an analgesic effect.

5. The achievement of the ability to sit up in infancy seems to be accompanied by a sense of control. When this developmental milestone is reached, the mere act of making an infant or child lie down usually results in crying and struggling to get up. As more force is used to hold the child down, the child increases efforts to get up, along with loud vocal protests. Recognizing lying down as a significant contributor to the child's distress enables one to avoid this position and create other strategies to ensure immobilization sufficient to allow safe completion of the procedure while reinforcing the child's sense of control. Two of the authors (BS, MB) researched and created alternative positioning techniques (Figs. 2-1 through 2-4). These create a secure, comforting, hugging hold with close physical contact with the parent or caretaker and ensure that the caregiver provides positive assistance, not negative restraint. A sitting position allows a sense of control and permits visualization of the parent's face. In all these positions immobilization of the extremity can be successful.

6. Toddlers can be helped through a procedure by using distraction techniques: looking at a kaleidoscope or pinwheel, watching pop-up books, or blowing bubbles.

7. Preschool children may also benefit from distraction techniques but are mature enough to more actively participate. Children who are 3 and older may benefit from active imagery: telling a story about how their favorite superhero would handle the pain. Alternatively, the child may wish to listen to a story. A popular use of imagery is the "magic glove," or "magic blanket." Preschoolers exhibit magical thinking; events happen just because they think them. The "magic glove" takes advantage of this developmental phenomenon. An imaginary glove is placed on the child's hand finger by finger. The child is told that the glove will lessen the pain of the needlestick. Because children have vivid imaginations, the power of suggestion holds great power. A magic blanket may work on other body parts where a glove may not fit, such as the thigh, back, or hip. Preschoolers may be given some power over their pain by instructing them to visualize a switch in their head, and then turn it off.

8. Older children will benefit from preparation and may participate in active imagery such as imagining sports, video games, or amusement park rides. In general school-age children are concrete thinkers. It may be beneficial to comment positively on some physical aspect of the child, for example, "Your muscles are very strong."

9. Relaxation training, similar to the Lamaze childbirth techniques, may be very helpful to adolescents. Progressive relaxation accompanied by slow deep

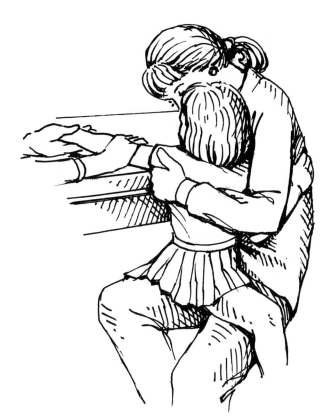

Figure 2–1. Immobilization for procedures can safely be accomplished by having the child sit facing the parent, encircled in a hug. Sitting up gives the child a sense of control and mastery. The child may watch the procedure if he or she wishes.

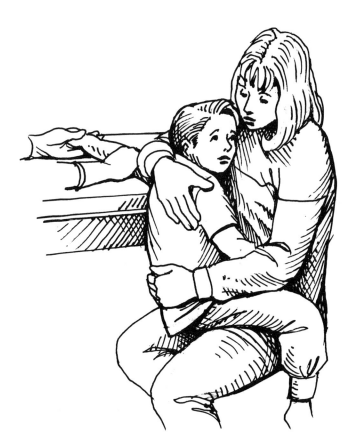

Figure 2–2. In the sitting position, the child has the choice to look away if he or she wishes.

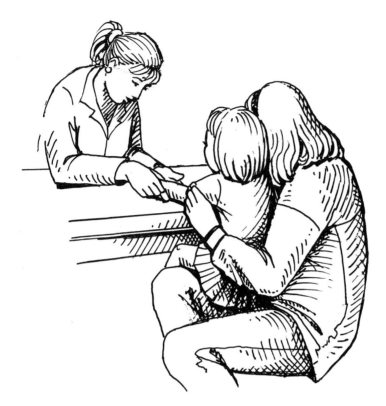

Figure 2–3. If the child cannot straddle the parent because of injuries or surgery, he or she may be positioned across the parent's knee.

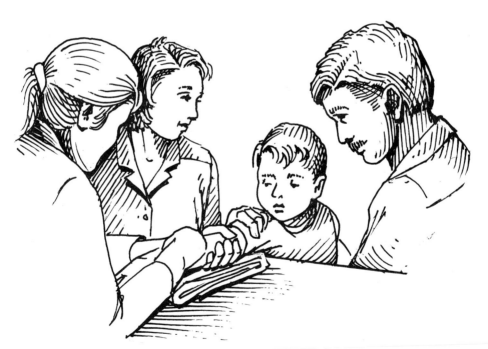

Figure 2–4. With the parent's support, and the assistance of another adult to immobilize the limb, even a 2-year-old can cooperate with procedures.

Table 2-2. **AGE-APPROPRIATE NONPHARMACOLOGIC STRATEGIES**

Age	Interventions	Age	Interventions
Neonate/Infant	Containment, swaddling Sucking, holding, rocking, rhythmic movements, soft voice, rapid rocking with patting and gradual slowing until calm	School-age	Distraction (video games, books) Imagery, relaxation, hypnosis Preparation, explanation Parental presence Music, TV
Toddler	Rocking Parental presence Distraction with bright movable objects, music Minimal restraint to allow movement Postprocedural play, massage		Biofeedback Active involvement, hand-holding
		Adolescent	Preparation and explanation Progressive relaxation Music (headphones) Self-hypnosis, imagery Choices, support person
Preschool	Distraction (pop-up books) Favorite stories Active imagery Parental presence Preprocedural and postprocedural play Modeling, preparation Choices, praise Blowing (bubbles or party-type blowers) Minimal restraint		

Parental presence is helpful at any age. Adolescents should be given a choice whether or not to have a parent present. Massage and the use of heat or cold may also be helpful in some situations for the older child.

breathing may lessen pain. In addition, the child may be encouraged to visualize himself or herself in a relaxing environment (the beach, a meadow, a spring rain).

10. When performing the procedure, talk in a quiet voice with a continuous description of the procedure. For example, "Now I am wiping your hand, it will feel cold, it will not hurt." Allow the child to express feelings. Use encouraging words for both the child and the parent. Praise the child (and parent) before, during, and after the procedure.

A few minutes invested in these nonpharmacologic strategies will reward all involved with huge dividends. The strategies will permit children to avoid suffering and experience mastery. In the era of health-care reform, these strategies are a wise choice: they are free, easily implemented, widely available, and perfectly safe.

References

Acute pain management: Operative or medical procedures and trauma. Clinical Practice Guidelines. Rockville, MD, Agency for Health Care Policy and Research, Public Health Service, US Department of Health and Human Services, 1992.

Amand KJS, McGrath PJ (eds). Pain in Neonates. New York, Elsevier Science Publishers, 1993.

Campos RG. Rocking and pacifiers: Two comforting interventions for heelstick pain. Res Nurs Health 17:321-331, 1994.

Campos RG. Soothing pain elicited distress in infants with swaddling and pacifiers. Child Dev 60:781-792, 1989.

Kachoyeanos MK, Friedhoff M. Cognitive and behavioral strategies to reduce children's pain. MCN Am J Matern Child Nurs 18:14-19, 1993.

McGrath PA. Pain in Children. New York, Guilford Press, 1990.

McGrath PA, Craig KD. Developmental and psychological factors in children's pain. Pediatr Clin North Am 36:823-836, 1989.

McGrath PA, McAlpine L. Psychologic perspectives on pediatric pain. J Pediatr 122:52-58, 1993.

Olness K. Hypnotherapy: A cyberphysiologic strategy in pain management. Pediatr Clin North Am 36:873-884, 1989.

Shapiro BS, Cohen DE, Covelman KW, et al. Experience of an Interdisciplinary Team. Pediatrics 88:1226-1232, 1991.

Schechter NL, Berde CB, Yaster M (eds). Pain in infants, children and adolescents. Baltimore, Williams and Wilkins, 1993.

CHAPTER 3

Celeste M. Marx

PROCEDURAL SEDATION AND ANALGESIA

Providing for the relief of anxiety and discomfort during painful medical and minor surgical procedures in children has the potential to be an adventure fraught with difficulty. The practitioner, desiring to use the safest of effective agents, may have had only anecdotal experience as a guide. Until recently, the medical literature contained few if any controlled evaluations of the many agents used in pediatrics that would allow comparison of their relative efficacy and safety. Widespread concern over the discrepancy between practice and research has led to the conduct and publication of a reasonable number of studies. Even so, most agents that have been evaluated have been studied in the context of laceration repair. This is a frequent procedure and one that many children tolerate well with appropriate local anesthesia and distraction techniques.

Because not all agents have been systematically compared in children, application of a number of maxims can facilitate safe and effective sedation and analgesia.

Conscious sedation should be considered as part of the care of children undergoing unpleasant or painful procedures. Not all children require sedation when appropriate preparation and support are provided. When a child must undergo repeated procedures, distress increases over the course of therapy and the need for sedation increases. Avoidance of a bad initial experience may help to prevent a cycle of anxiety and distress behaviors, which compromises the safety of the procedure. Optimal sedation cannot be expected to compensate for inadequate educational preparation, insensitive emotional support, inadequate staffing, or problems with technique (such as omitting local anesthetics).

Sedative response in children is frequently less than completely predictable. Dosages of sedative or analgesic agents must be individualized. Safe use of any agent requires knowledge of usual onset, peak, and duration of action and of side effects (Table 3-1). The patient should receive additional incremental doses only after an appropriate time has elapsed to assess the efficacy of the agent (onset) but not after waiting so long that the partial sedative effect achieved after the first dose is lost. This helps to prevent excessive "stacking" of doses and overshooting the desired therapeutic endpoint. Unfortunately, maximal doses, as identified in Table 3-1 have not been systematically determined. Individual children may require higher doses to achieve sedation and may tolerate them well. A maximal safe total dose in a given period should be identified by sedation protocol, based on the population to be sedated, the procedure to be performed, and the availability of support or resuscitative personnel.

In general, polypharmacy (the use of multiple agents) should be avoided. Polypharmacy frequently produces unpredictable additive efficacy and results in synergistic effects on respiratory depression (for those agents for which this is a side effect). Varying combinations or redosing strategies (altered time until the initial dose is reinforced or a second agent added) need to be evaluated like new agents, as has recently been reported for the combination of sufentanil and midazolam by intranasal application. In some cases, combinations of agents are rational and lead to reduced side effects (e.g., ketamine combined with atropine to prevent hypersalivation). Matching agents with disparate side effects may allow adequate efficacy with improved safety; however, any advantage should be established by clinical data. Re-evaluation of time-honored or newer combinations still in common use (meperidine-promethazine-chlorpromazine or meperidine-midazolam) has revealed substantial risks of cardiovascular and respiratory side effects, greater than commonly assumed. Part of this recognition may be due to adherence to recommendations for more consistent monitoring of all children being sedated.

Sedatives must be used in an appropriate setting. Regardless of where the procedure is performed and who supervises the sedation. A trained observer (in addition to the person performing the procedure) should monitor the child during sedation, the procedure, and the recovery period, recording observations until the child is back to his or her neurologic baseline of alertness. The observer must be able to assess vital signs, level of consciousness, depth and frequency of respiration, airway condition, and need for ventilatory support. Pulse oximetry is superior to visual observation for color in detecting subclinical and incipient changes in cardiorespiratory status. The sedation, procedural, and recovery area(s) should have oxygen, breathing circuit, and suction devices available. Resuscitation medications and equipment must be immediately available, along with personnel trained in their use. Attention should be paid to appropriate nothing-by-mouth guidelines (3 to 4 hours for planned procedures) whenever possible.

Personnel and equipment for the procedure should be prepared and available to act as soon as adequate sedation is achieved. Failed response to voice, positioning, or nailbed squeeze may be appropriate endpoints for determining the depth of sedation, depending on the procedure to be performed. This is particularly important when rapid-acting agents are used in a setting in which sedatives with slow onset and recovery have been routinely chosen in the past. Choice of agents with rapid onset results not only in more efficient sedation and greater convenience but also in finer titration of the dosage to individual patient requirement, as any necessary repeated dosage is usually not given before the full effect of the prior dose is evaluated.

Short-acting agents may need to be repeated to sustain adequate sedation for protracted procedures. Incremental partial doses (i.e., one-third to one-half the usual effective dose given initially) given before full recovery occurs generally allow satisfactory sedation without excessive prolongation of recovery. If too much time elapses in assessing the inadequacy of the initial dose, higher total doses may be required to finally achieve sedation, increasing the risk of side effects and sedation failure. Conversely, if the repeated dose is given before the first dose has had time to achieve full effect, an excessive sedative effect may be seen. Repeated doses should not be given until the peak effect of the prior dose has been expected or observed (see Table 3–1). Although consistent experience with a single agent or regimen will help in predicting when the best time to redose is, pediatric patients vary substantially in their individual responses to a given regimen.

Cardiovascular side effects (altered heart rate or blood pressure) may occur together, regardless of state of sedation. Abnormal vital signs may be most easily recognized by trained personnel and facilitated by use of age-specific normal charts. A plan should be formulated for assessing the airway and patient position and for

Text continued on page 23

Table 3–1. DOSAGES AND PHARMACOLOGIC FEATURES OF SEDATIVES

Agent	Route	Dose	Maximum Dose	Onset	Peak	Duration	Side Effects	Comments
Analgesic Sedatives								
Opioid Analgesics	*Generally provide conscious sedation in doses used for procedural sedation*							
Morphine	IV	0.05–0.15 mg/kg over 5 minutes	10 mg	10–20 min	20–30 min	1 hr	Respiratory depression (depth reduced before rate)	Excellent sedation and analgesia
	IM	0.05–0.2 mg/kg	10 mg	15–30 min	30–90 min	1–2 hr	Bradycardia, tachycardia (meperidine)	Effects fully reversible with naloxone
	PO	0.3–0.5 mg/kg	30 mg	20–30 min	45–60 min	1–2 hr	Hypotension (due to histamine release and venodilation)	Careful dose titration generally producing a cooperative patient with acceptable respiration
Meperidine (Demerol)	IV	1–2 mg/kg over 5 min	100 mg	10 min		1 hr	Nausea, vomiting	
	IM	1–2.25 mg/kg	112.5 mg	15–20 min	1 hr	1–2 hr	High doses:	
	PO	2–4 mg/kg	200 mg	15–20 min	1 hr	1–2 hr	Narcosis—coma, respiratory depression, constricted pupils, hypotension; seizures (especially morphine in newborns)	
Fentanyl (Sublimaze)	IV	0.5–1 µg/kg q 5 min over 3–5 min	5 µg/kg	3–5 min	5–15 min	20 min	All previous side effects, with less risk of histamine release and cardiovascular changes but greater risk of chest wall rigidity (partially) reversible with naloxone; reversible with neuromuscular blockade; recurrent narcosis (4 hr postsurgery) seen after use of high doses	Fentanyl derivatives generally short acting and useful for brief procedures
	TM (Lollipop)	5–15 µg/kg	400 µg	30 min		30–60 min	Transmucosal fentanyl associated with frequent vomiting and pruritus (20–33%)	
Sufentanil (Sufenta)	IN	0.5–0.75 µg/kg				30–60 min		

Nonopioid Analgesics *Provide analgesia to dissociative anesthesia depending on dose; monitor like deep sedation*

Nonanalgesic Sedatives

Benzodiazepines *Generally provide conscious sedation*

Drug	Route	Dose	Max dose	Onset	Peak	Duration	Cautions	Comments
Alfentanil (Alfenta)	IV	1.5–3 μg/kg over 3–5 min q 5 min	9 μg/kg	<5 min		<15–20 min		Analgesia equivalent to morphine with good sedation
Nalbuphine (Nubain)	IV	0.1–.15 mg/kg over 3–5 min	20 mg	<5 min		20–60 min	Limited respiratory depression allowing safer titration to adequate sedation; not habit forming; lesser effect to constrict sphincter of Oddi	
Ketamine (Ketalar)	IV	0.5–2 mg/kg over 1 min	100 mg	1 min	5–10 min	10–20 min	Hypersalivation, preventable with atropine 0.1 mg/kg mixed into ketamine dose	In addition to high-quality sedation and analgesia, produces amnesia for procedure
	IM	3–7 mg/kg		7 min	10 min	10–40 min	Catecholamine release: increased blood pressure, heart rate, and respiratory rate; increased muscle tone; uncommon emesis; rare laryngospasm. Emergence delirium in 10–33% of children during arousal; avoidance of excessive stimuli during arousal; preventable with concomitant use of benzodiazepine, which increases duration of action slightly	
	PO	5–10 mg/kg		30–45 min		10–40 min		
	IN	5 mg/kg		<7 min		10–40 min		
Diazepam (Valium)	IV	0.1–0.2 mg/kg over 2–3 min	10 mg	5 min	10 min	30–60 min	Respiratory depression (related to both dose and rate of injection)	Variable-quality sedation; some children become agitated ("paradoxic agitation"); provides anxiolysis, anterograde amnesia; good muscle relaxation; reversible with flumazenil (see Table 3–2)
	PO	0.2–0.5 mg/kg		60–90 min		60 min	Painful injection (diazepam, lorazepam)	
	PR	0.2–0.4 mg/kg (use IV solution)		10 min	10–90 min	20–100 min		

Table continued on following page

Table 3–1. DOSAGES AND PHARMACOLOGIC FEATURES OF SEDATIVES *Continued*

Agent	Route	Dose	Maximum Dose	Onset	Peak	Duration	Side Effects	Comments
Nonanalgesic Sedatives *Continued*								
Lorazepam (Ativan)	IV	0.05–0.1 mg/kg	2 mg	<5 min	25–30 min	30–60 min (mild sedation up to 8 hr)	Alcohol/propylene glycol diluent may be cardiac depressant (diazepam, lorazepam)	May cause paradoxical agitation.
	IM	0.05–0.1 mg/kg		15–30 min				
	PO	0.05–0.1 mg/kg (may give IV solution PO)		10–60 min				
Midazolam (Versed)	IV	0.05 mg/kg over 2 min every 5 min	0.2 mg/kg	1–5 min	10 min	30–60 min		May cause paradoxical agitation.
	IM	0.1–0.2 mg/kg		15 min	30–60 min	2 hr		
	PO	0.5–0.75 mg/kg children <5 yr; 0.3–0.5 mg/kg children >5 yr	15 mg	20–30 min	1 hr	1–1.5 hr		
	PR	0.3–0.7 mg/kg		20–30 min	30 min–1 hr	1–2 hr		
	IN	0.2–0.25 mg/kg over 15 sec; may repeat × 1 in 5–15 min		5 min	10–30 min	60 min		
Barbiturates *Generally provide excellent sedation with moderate risk of deep sedation*								
Pentobarbital (Nembutal) or secobarbital (Seconal)	IV	1–2 mg/kg over 3–5 min every 10 min up to 5 mg/kg	100 mg	30 sec	1 min	15–60 min	Hypotension (risk may be reduced by IV infusion over 3–5 min) Apnea and laryngospasm occur occasionally (reduce risk by injection at <50 mg/min or 1 mg/kg/min, generally over 3–5 min)	Rapid sedation of high quality; contributes to easily titrated level of sedation
	IM	2–6 mg/kg	200 mg	15–20 min	30–60 min	1–4 hr		
	PO/PR	2–6 mg/kg		15–60 min		1–4 hr		
Methohexital (Brevital)	IV	0.75–2 mg/kg	200 mg	<30 sec	30–40 sec	7–10 min	Hypotension, respiratory depression, laryngospasm	
	IM	5–10 mg/kg		5 min		1–1.5 hr		
	PR	20–25 mg/kg		6–10 min		20 min–1.5 hr	Occasional vomiting	

Drug	Route	Dose	Maximum dose	Onset	Peak	Duration	Side effects	Comments
Thiopental (Pentothal)	IV	4–6 mg/kg	500 mg	0.5–1 min		5–10 min	Hypotension, cardiac and respiratory depression, apnea, laryngospasm	
	PR	25 mg/kg; may repeat 12.5 mg/kg in 10–15 min if needed	1.5 g	10 min		20 min–5 hr		
Other Sedatives								
Chloral hydrate (Noctec)	PO or PR	50–125 mg/kg (50–75 mg/kg, may repeat in 30 min)	125 mg/kg or 2 g	30–60 min		1–8 hr	Rare apnea; rare laryngospasm	Provides conscious sedation; <50 mg/kg greatly increases risk of sedation failure; slow-onset limits ability to titrate dosage; better for noninvasive procedures
Propofol (Diprivan)	IV	0.5–2 mg/kg over 3–5 min		<30 sec	1 min	10–20 min	With higher dose, apnea may be seen in 20% of children; Hypotension (up to 10%); Bradycardia	Provides deep but very brief sedation unless infused; highly effective
Combination Sedatives								
"DPT Cocktail" (Demerol, Phenergan, Thorazine)	IM or IV slow infusion	Meperidine 1–2.5 mg/kg; Promethazine 0.5–1 mg/kg; Chlorpromazine 0.5–1 mg/kg	100 mg; 25 mg; 25 mg	30 min	45 min	1–2 hr	Not recommended, owing to frequent cardiovascular and respiratory side effects and protracted recovery (mean 2–4.5 hr)	All agents are suitable for controlled infusion over not less than 15–20 min; partially reversible with naloxone
Sufentanil-Midazolam (Sufenta-Versed)	IN	0.75 µg/kg; 0.2 mg/kg as slow stream from needle without syringe		20 min		50 min	Decline in blood pressure, respiratory depression (as earlier for each agent)	Combination reported to be more effective than same dose of either agent given alone; reversible with naloxone plus flumazenil
Topical Anesthetics	*May have central nervous system toxicity in excessive doses*							
Lidocaine	INJ	Varies with procedure; do not draw up more than maximum dose (1% solution = 10 mg/ml)	4.5 mg/kg in 2-hr period	45–90 sec		10–25 min	Sedation; agitation, seizures hypotension, heart block	Pain on injection can be reduced by buffering solution with 8.4% sodium bicarbonate (1 ml to 9 ml lidocaine)

Table continued on following page

Table 3–1. DOSAGES AND PHARMACOLOGIC FEATURES OF SEDATIVES *Continued*

Agent	Route	Dose	Maximum Dose	Onset	Peak	Duration	Side Effects	Comments
Topical Anesthetics *Continued*								
Lidocaine-Prilocaine (EMLA)	TOP	2.5 g/10 cm skin	Maximum skin area of application: 10 kg: 100 cm^2 10–20 kg: 600 cm^2 20 kg: 2000 cm^2	45 min–1 hr		1 hr after removal	Local skin blanching or irritation; rare methemoglobinemia	Does not reduce success of vascular cannulation; may be left under dressing up to 4 hr; not for infants less than 3 mo old
Tetracaine-Adrenaline-Cocaine ("TAC") (tetracaine 0.5%; adrenaline 1:2000; cocaine 11.8%)	TOP	3–5 ml of solution per each 3-cm length of wound (sterile gauze may be soaked and placed in wound)	0.09 ml/kg	10–20 min		20–30 min	Systemic cocaine toxicity may be seen, including disorientation, seizures, and death in excessive amounts or if ingested (by licking or dripping into mouth)	Do not apply to mucous membranes, eyes, or areas with end arteriolar blood supply (digits, nose, earlobes, penis)
Lidocaine-Adrenaline-Tetracaine (LAT) (tetracaine 0.5%; adrenaline 1:2000; lidocaine 4%)	TOP	3–5 ml of solution per each 3-cm length of wound	4.5 mg/kg Lidocaine in 2-hr period	15–20 min		20–30 min		

IV, Intravenous; IM, intramuscular; PO, per os; IN, intranasal; PR, per rectum; TM, transmucosal; TOP, topical.

providing stimulation to arouse the patient. Administration of fluid or medications (i.e., atropine for bradycardia, antidotes for benzodiazepines or narcotics) should be formulated in advance as part of the sedation protocol, with the medications readily available on the resuscitation cart or medication area.

Ventilatory side effects (respiratory depression, apnea) may occur at any time after administration of central nervous system active drugs. Although most commonly expected after rapid administration of intravenous respiratory depressant agents, these effects may be most profound after the stimulation of the procedure is complete and the patient is positioned to recover. Altered response to carbon dioxide persists many hours longer than effective sedation *and* recovery to full alertness, for most narcotic, benzodiazepine, and barbiturate agents. Agents used in combination generally have synergistic (more than additive) effects on ventilatory response. Because this effect is not easily predicted by age or habitus, all patients should be carefully monitored for respiratory effects at least through complete central nervous system recovery. With morphine and meperidine, altered response to carbon dioxide persists for more than 4 hours after the end of sedative effects. After the use of meperidine-promethazine-chlorpromazine (DPT), cardiorespiratory events have been reported as late as 14 hours after sedation. Certain children may be at particular risk of respiratory side effects. Developmentally delayed children may have a higher risk of airway compromise during sedation, particularly those with poor oral-pharyngeal muscle tone or abnormal jaw position or size. Children with cardiac or chronic lung disorders may also be at higher risk for adverse effects, as are those with renal or hepatic dysfunction. Children who have experienced respiratory depression and required narcotic or benzodiazepine reversal agents will need to be monitored for the end of the antidote effect and several hours thereafter, to reduce the risk of recurrent respiratory depression.

Cardiovascular and respiratory side effects occur regardless of the route of administration of the agent. Rapid intravenous administration usually reduces the time of onset of a medication, and may produce greater central nervous system (CNS) effects (greater efficacy) with a higher risk of side effects related to brain drug concentrations. Use of administration routes other than intravenous (IV) usually results in somewhat slower transit of the drug to the brain. Unfortunately, erratic or incomplete absorption is typical (noting the higher doses required by alternate routes). Use of oral, rectal, intranasal, and transmucosal agents has increased with availability of highly lipophilic agents (such as fentanyl, alfentanil, sufentanil, midazolam). Route does not define safety. Patients require the same monitoring, regardless of the route of administration of the potent sedative or analgesic agent. An intramuscular route is not a humane choice when an IV line is available and when the selected agents may be given at a controlled rate of injection. Not only are some agents unreliably and slowly absorbed after intramuscular administration but it is psychologically unreasonable to begin preparation for a procedure by inflicting the pain of injection. Finally, local or topical anesthetics (including buffered lidocaine, tetracaine-adrenaline-cocaine [TAC]) may have CNS effects as well.

Fear of side effects need not lead the practitioner to avoid sedation or administer insufficient dosages. The effects of the agents in most common use for pediatric procedures (narcotics and benzodiazepines) are fully reversible. Even though use of low doses does not prevent side effects of greatest concern (e.g., laryngospasm, cardiovascular effects), it does prevent efficacy fairly reliably. In underdosing, children often become progressively more disinhibited and uncooperative. Interestingly, paradoxic agitation is often seen with use of high doses of benzodiazepines.

The specific agent to be used in a given procedure should be determined by

Table 3–2. **REASONABLE SEDATIVE CHOICES FOR PROCEDURES OF VARIOUS LENGTH AND DEGREE OF PAIN INDUCED***

Procedure	Usually Effective Agents (listed in order of preference)	Procedure	Usually Effective Agents (listed in order of preference)
Painless diagnostic study requiring cooperation	Infant: Benzodiazepine (IN/PO/ PR/IV) Chloral hydrate (PO/PR) Thiopental (PR) Child: Benzodiazepine (PO) Pentobarbital (IM/IV) Propofol (IV)	Laceration repair in uncooperative patient	Benzodiazepine (PO/IN/PR) Thiopental (PR) Ketamine (PO)
Lumbar puncture in cooperative patient	Distraction techniques plus buffered lidocaine	Protracted or facial laceration repair	Ketamine (IM/IV)† Fentanyl (IV) Midazolam (PO/IN/IV)
Lumbar puncture in uncooperative patient	Morphine (IV/IM) or meperidine (IV/IM) or fentanyl (IV) Benzodiazepine (IV/IN/PO)	Incision and drainage of abscess	Fentanyl (IV) Ketamine (IM)
Bone marrow aspiration or biopsy in uncooperative patient	Ketamine (IV/IM/PO)†	Extraction of foreign body	Ketamine (IM/IV) Thiopental (PR)
		Sexual abuse examination	Benzodiazepine (PO/IN) Fentanyl (IV) Ketamine (IV/IM/PO)
Laceration repair in cooperative or distractable patient	Distraction techniques plus buffered lidocaine TAC or LAT	Fracture reduction	Ketamine (IM/IV) Fentanyl (IV) or Morphine (IV/IM) or Meperidine (IV/IM) Benzodiazapine (IV)

IV, Intravenous; IM, intramuscular; SC, subcutaneous; PO, per os; IN, intranasal; TAC, tetracaine/adrenaline/cocaine topical solution (see text).

*Appropriateness for a given setting will depend on availability of personnel and equipment to manage adverse reactions and a specific protocol for monitoring safety.

†Ketamine should be given with atropine to prevent excessive salivation and with benzodiazepine to reduce risk of psychotomimetic reactions.

Table 3–3. **ANTIDOTES FOR OVERSEDATION: SEDATIVE "REVERSERS"**

Agent	Reversers	Dosage	Timing	Comments
Flumazenil (Romazicon)	Benzodiazepines (Diazepam, Lorazepam, Midazolam, and others)	0.01 mg/kg over 30 sec; may repeat every minute up to 1 mg (usual dose 0.025 mg/kg)	Onset: 1–3 min Peak: 6–10 min Duration: 20–60 min	Use in benzodiazepine-dependent patients can precipitate seizures; nausea and vomiting may be seen; use indicates longer, rather than shorter, postsedation observation.
Naloxone (Narcan)	Opioid agents (narcotics: morphine, meperidine, fentanyl, alfentanil, sufentanil, and others)	Titration to reverse toxicity only: 0.001–0.002 mg/kg over 30 sec every 2–3 min until respiratory rate, heart rate, blood pressure, or level of consciousness response is achieved Full reversal: 0.01 mg/ kg IV, IM, SC, or IO over 30 sec; may double every 2–3 min until 0.1 mg/kg	Onset: 2 min Duration: 30–45 min	Use in opioid-dependent patient may precipitate severe withdrawal (including dysphoria, seizures, muscle cramps, tearing, rhinorrhea, and diarrhea). Use indicates longer, rather than shorter, postsedation observation.

SC, Subcutaneous; IO, intraosseous; IV, intravenous; IM, intramuscular.

the pharmacologic effects desired and characteristics of its onset and recovery. When a local anesthetic alone will not blunt the pain from the procedure, an analgesic agent (opioids or ketamine) should be chosen. It is not unreasonable to consider administration of a nonsteroidal anti-inflammatory agent to the child waiting for the painful procedure. These agents (acetaminophen, ibuprofen, naproxen, or ketorolac) may reduce pain and, indirectly, anxiety in approaching the procedure. If anxiety is a major component of the child's distress (evident even before the procedure is undertaken) benzodiazepine anxiolytics are desirable. Benzodiazepines have the additional advantage of anterograde amnesia, in which nothing is remembered after the time of administration of the drug but instructions and preparation before the procedure are retained. Barbiturates, ketamine, and chloral hydrate have the advantage of preserving the cough reflex and not increasing the risk of aspiration. These agents with a preserved cough reflex during sedation may rarely be associated with laryngospasm, so unnecessary examination of the airway should be avoided. This may be disadvantageous in certain procedures but is usually not a barrier to bronchoscopy, in which lidocaine is applied to the trachea. When a very unpleasant procedure is to be undertaken, when the patient would really prefer not to be present (sexual abuse examination, dental examination in the developmentally disabled, burn debridement), ketamine may offer the unique advantage of dissociative anesthetic/analgesic effects, in which patients do not associate the procedural events with anything happening to their body. Ketamine is also desirable when a motionless patient is preferred (e.g., foreign body removal) (some may be so motionless as to be rigid). Appropriate sedative regimens for certain types of procedures are provided in Table 3–2.

After the maximal predetermined dosage of a usually effective agent has been tried, a second agent may be added, providing the initial agent has been well tolerated. Because the additional effect may be unpredictable, it is safest for this to be a fully reversible agent (narcotic or benzodiazepine). If excessive effects occur, the reversal agent may be given to reverse the undesired effect. Anesthesiologists titrate the dose of naloxone or flumazenil by giving very small incremental doses (Table 3–3) to achieve reversal of cardiovascular or respiratory side effects without loss of the sedative effect whenever possible.

After maximal dosage of the single or simple combination agents has been tried, or side effects encountered, anesthesiologist consultation may be the safest approach for the apparently difficult-to-sedate patient. The armamentarium of the anesthesiologist includes potent agents that are nearly always successful and whose side effects may be readily managed by the anesthesiologist in a controlled setting.

Discharge instructions to the child's caregivers should include postsedation instructions. This may include delaying the next feeding or meal for 1 to 2 hours to reduce the risk of postsedation vomiting; avoidance of unsupervised play or activities requiring care, coordination, or concentration; and supervised baths or machinery use for up to 8 hours.

AIRWAY AND BREATHING

CHAPTER 4

Michele Walsh-Sukys

BAG AND MASK VENTILATION

INDICATIONS

1. Apnea
2. Respiratory failure

CONTRAINDICATIONS

1. Neonates suspected of having a congenital diaphragmatic hernia should be intubated in the trachea and ventilated to avoid distending the bowel.
2. Relative: Patients with severe facial trauma may be difficult or impossible to ventilate.

EQUIPMENT

1. Mask: Sized to cover nose and mouth
2. Ventilating bag
   a. Anesthesia bag (flow inflating): Bag is deflated when not in use; inflates only when an air or oxygen source is connected to it (Fig. 4-1)
   b. Self-inflating bag: Remains inflated at all times; does not require a compressed gas source, and therefore is portable (Fig. 4-2): unable to deliver oxygen concentrations exceeding 0.4 unless reservoir attached
3. Oxygen source
4. Optional but recommended equipment
   a. Pressure gauge

PROCEDURE

1. Assemble and test bag by occluding patient outflow with the palm of your hand. Deliver several "breaths," testing that the bag delivers desired pressure, and that the overpressurization valve opens. If using an anesthesia-style bag, ensure that the bag inflates when a seal is obtained.
2. Check patient's position to ensure that the airway is open. The neck should be slightly extended, with the nose in a "sniffing" position.
3. Position the mask to cover both the nose and the mouth, and obtain a seal

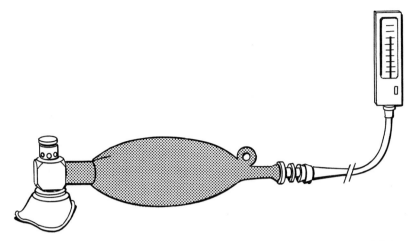

Figure 4–1. An anesthesia resuscitation bag requires a constant gas source to inflate.

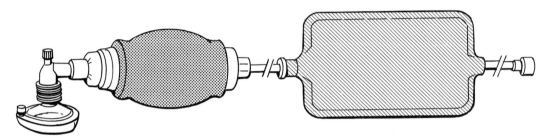

Figure 4–2. A self-inflating bag does not require a gas source and is therefore portable.

Hook middle finger under chin

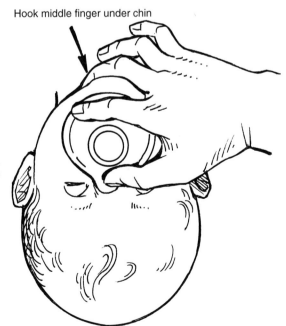

Figure 4–3. Properly positioned face mask that is held in place by one hand using the thumb and ring finger. The third finger ensures a seal by hooking under the chin.

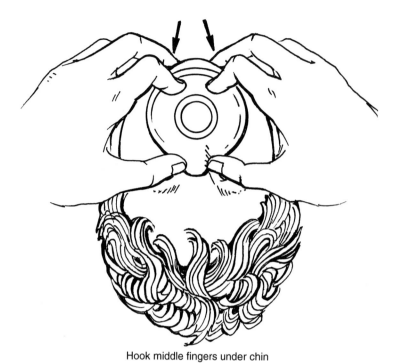

Hook middle fingers under chin

Figure 4–4. A face mask may be held in place with two hands to ensure that a complete seal is obtained. A second individual provides bag ventilation.

Figure 4–5. When positioning the mask, care must be taken to avoid placing over the eyes, which may injure the globes, or over the submental region, which may produce airway occlusion.

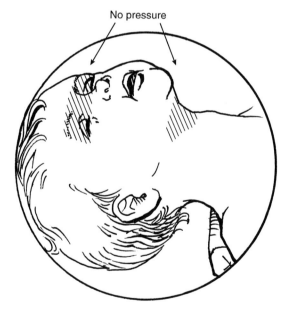

No pressure

between mask and face. It may be helpful to begin by placing the mask over the chin, and rocking it back on to the face. The mask is usually held in place with the thumb and index finger on the mask, while the third or ring finger holds the chin in the mask (Fig. 4-3). Alternatively, the mask may be positioned using two hands surrounding the mask while hooking the middle fingers underneath the chin (Fig. 4-4). Care must be taken to avoid placement of the mask over the eyes or over the submental region (Fig. 4-5). Check for adequacy of seal by observing for chest rise while delivering three to four breaths.

4. Ventilate at the rate appropriate for age.

Age	Rate (Breaths per Min)	Mnemonics
Newborn	30	Every 2 sec
Toddler	20	Every 3 sec
Older child	15	Every 4 sec

5. Ventilate with the lowest pressure that achieves chest rise.
6. In older children, bag and mask ventilation should be accompanied by cricoid pressure (also known as Sellick maneuver) to occlude the esophagus (see Fig. 7-1).

COMPLICATIONS

1. Inability to ventilate because of inadequate seal or torn bag (the most common place for a leak to occur is between the cheek and the bridge of the nose)
2. Overpressurization due either to overenthusiastic bagging or to malfunction of the overpressurization valve
3. Injury to the eye globes from malposition of the mask or from a mask that is too large and placed over the orbits
4. Airway obstruction owing to mask malposition over the submental area rather than on the mandible, or owing to head malposition

References

Bloom RS, Cropley C. *Textbook of Neonatal Resuscitation.* Dallas, American Heart Association and American Academy of Pediatrics, 1987.
Chameides L (ed). *Textbook of Pediatric Advanced Life Support.* Dallas, American Heart Association and American Academy of Pediatrics, 1988.

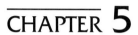
Michele Walsh-Sukys

PLACEMENT OF ORAL AIRWAY

INDICATIONS

1. Neonatal
   a. Bilateral choanal atresia: Infants are obligate nasal breathers; therefore, if both nares are obstructed, severe distress will be present at birth. Choanal atresia results from a congenital blockage of one or both of the posterior nares by either a membrane or a bone.
   b. Airway obstruction due to either small jaw (Pierre Robin syndrome) or large tongue (Beckwith-Wiedemann syndrome, Down's syndrome)
2. Pediatric
   a. Blockage of airway by tongue caused by altered mental status

EQUIPMENT

1. Oral airway with size appropriate for age. The proper size may be estimated by holding the airway against the patient's cheek with the flange portion at the lip. The curved tip should reach to the angle of the jaw.
2. Gloves

PROCEDURE

1. Select appropriate size airway. The airway should comfortably fit over the tongue.
2. Put on gloves.
3. Open the mouth (Fig. 5-1). Lift the tongue with a tongue depressor and gently insert the airway over the tongue. In older pediatric patients one may insert the airway with the curve facing sideways and then rotate the airway over the tongue. In neonates this maneuver is rarely needed.

COMPLICATIONS

1. Obstruction of airway by tongue if airway is too small
2. Laceration of tongue or palate if airway is too large

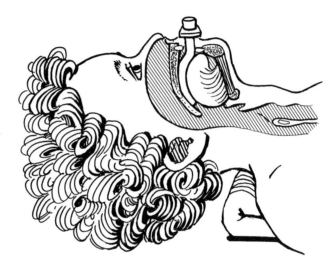

Figure 5–1. A properly positioned oral airway reaches the base of the tongue.

CHAPTER 6

Michele Walsh-Sukys

NASAL AIRWAY

INDICATIONS

1. Pediatric: Protection of airway in patient with an impaired ability to maintain airway but who is sufficiently awake and may not tolerate an oral airway

EQUIPMENT

1. Nasal airway: Available in sizes from 12 to 36 Fr. The appropriate diameter and length vary by age. The airway should be easily admitted into the nares, without causing blanching of the alae nasae. The proper length can be estimated by measuring the distance from the tip of the nose to the tragus of the ear.
2. Gloves

TECHNIQUE

1. Lubricate the airway.
2. Gently insert through a nostril and advance in a posterior direction perpendicular to the plane of the face (Fig. 6–1).

COMPLICATIONS

1. Laceration of nasopharynx
2. Occlusion of narrow diameter airways by mucus or blood

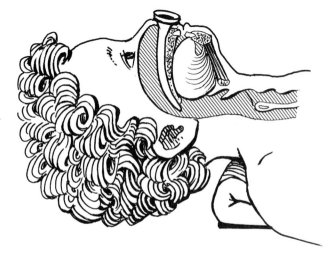

Figure 6–1. A nasal airway trumpet will easily pass into the nares if the proper size has been chosen.

CHAPTER 7

Michele Walsh-Sukys

OROTRACHEAL INTUBATION

INDICATIONS

1. Prolonged positive pressure ventilation
2. Ineffective bag and mask ventilation
3. Altered consciousness, which may prohibit the patient from protecting the airway
4. Relief of critical upper airway obstruction

EQUIPMENT

1. Laryngoscope
2. Blades
    a. Straight blades are preferred in neonates:
        (1) Miller size 0 for preterm
        (2) Miller size 1 for term
    b. Curved blades are preferred in older children and have a flange on the left side designed to prevent the tongue from obscuring the view.
    c. In older children the correct blade length can be approximated by the distance from the corner of the mouth to the tragus.
3. Endotracheal tube: Appropriate for age and size (Table 7-1)
4. Endotracheal tube stylet

TECHNIQUE

1. Place the patient in the "sniffing" position (nose pointing vertically), unless there is suspicion of head or neck injury in which case the neutral position must be maintained using manual in-line cervical immobilization.
2. Preoxygenate and/or ventilate the patient with bag and mask ventilation while applying cricoid pressure to occlude the esophagus (also known as the Sellick maneuver) (Fig. 7-1).
3. Hold the laryngoscope in the left hand (regardless of which of the intubator's hands are dominant).
4. Insert the blade into the mouth along the right side of the tongue. Once the blade is advanced to the base of the tongue, the tongue is gently moved by sliding the blade from the right side to the middle. This creates an unobstructed channel in the right one third of the mouth through which the endotracheal tube will be passed (Fig. 7-2).
5. When a curved blade is used, its tip is placed in the vallecula above the

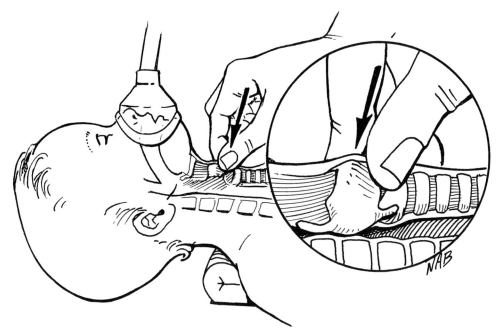

Figure 7–1. Gentle pressure on the cricothyroid membrane will occlude the esophagus and minimize gastric distention produced by bag and mask ventilation.

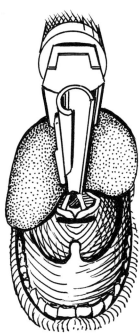

Figure 7–2. The laryngoscope is inserted to the base of the tongue, and the tongue is gently shifted away from the right side, creating a channel through which the endotracheal tube is passed.

Table 7–1. **ENDOTRACHEAL TUBE SIZES AND DEPTH OF INSERTION**

Age Group	Tube Size (ID mm)	Depth of Insertion (cm) (Lip to Midtrachea)
Newborn		
<1.0 kg	2.5 uncuffed	7
1.0–2.0 kg	3.0 uncuffed	8
2.0–3.0 kg	3.5 uncuffed	9
>3.0	4.0 uncuffed	10
1–6 mo	4.0 uncuffed	12
1 yr	4.0, 4.5 uncuffed	12
2–3 yr	4.5 uncuffed	14
4–5 yr	5.0 uncuffed	16
6–7 yr	5.5 uncuffed	16
8–9 yr	6.0 cuffed or uncuffed	18
10–11 yr	6.5 cuffed or uncuffed	18
12–13 yr	7.0 cuffed	20
14–15 yr	7.5 cuffed	22

epiglottis (Fig. 7–3). When a straight blade is used, its tip is placed below the epiglottis and above the glottic opening (Fig. 7–4).

6. Once positioned, traction is placed upward along the axis of the handle. This should create an "up and away" effort, which the intubator may feel in the upper arm musculature. Care must be taken to avoid using the upper gum or teeth as a fulcrum against which the laryngoscope is rocked back toward the intubator.

7. The tracheal tube is inserted from the right corner of the mouth to avoid obscuring the view of the glottic space (Fig. 7–5). The intubator should be able to visualize the tube as it passes between the vocal cords. The glottic marker (if present) is placed at the level of the vocal cords. Alternatively, the depth of insertion can be determined from Table 7-1. Cuffed endotracheal tubes are inserted so that the cuff is just below the vocal cords. Each attempt at intubation should be limited to 20 seconds to prevent hypoxemia.

8. Proper positioning of the endotracheal tube must be determined immediately by (1) auscultating equal breath sounds over each chest wall, (2) observing chest rise with bag inflation, (3) observing presence of mist in the endotracheal tube during expiration, and (4) noting the absence of breath sounds over the stomach. If these criteria cannot be confirmed, the endotracheal tube must be removed and bag and mask ventilation resumed.

9. Confirm endotracheal tube position with a radiograph.

10. In most patients it is desirable to have a small air leak around the endotracheal tube, as this reduces the likelihood of airway injury related to the use of an endotracheal tube that is too large. If the tube is cuffed, inflate the cuff with the volume indicated on the endotracheal tube.

11. Cut endotracheal tube so that no more than 4 cm remains between lip and adapter. This will reduce dead space and airway resistance, which could contribute to carbon dioxide retention.

12. Fix orotracheal tube to the patient's upper lip using tape (Fig. 7-6) or an external fixation device (Logan's bow support, modified umbilical cord clamp, or commercially available fixation device).

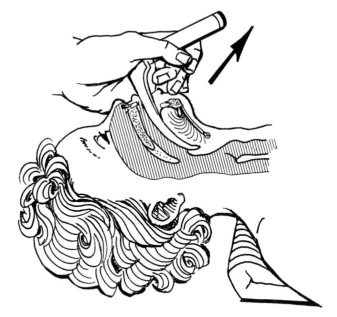

Figure 7–3. If a curved blade is used, its tip is inserted into the vallecula above the epiglottis.

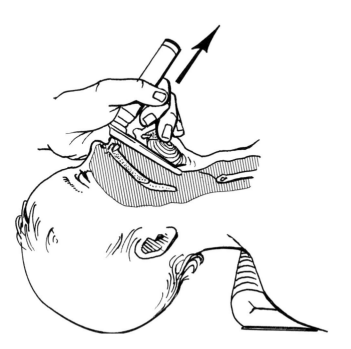

Figure 7–4. If a straight blade is used, its tip is inserted below the epiglottis.

CHAPTER 8

Michele Walsh-Sukys

NASOTRACHEAL INTUBATION

INDICATIONS

1. Long-term tracheal intubation (adult patients report that nasotracheal intubation is more comfortable than oral intubation)
2. Surgery of the face and mouth
3. Intubation in which oral intubation is made difficult by anomalies of the face, mouth, or jaw

CONTRAINDICATION

1. Trauma to midface.

EQUIPMENT

1. Laryngoscope
2. Blades
   a. Straight blades preferred in neonates
      (1) Miller size 0 for preterm
      (2) Miller size 1 for term
   b. Curved blades are preferred in older children and have a flange on the left side designed to prevent the tongue from obscuring the view
3. Endotracheal tube: Appropriate for age and size
4. Magill forceps

TECHNIQUE

1. If intubation is performed in an emergency, orotracheal intubation is the preferred method. Placement may then be electively converted to the nasotracheal position.
2. Placement under direct visualization
   a. Place the patient in the "sniffing" position.
   b. Insert a lubricated endotracheal tube through the nostril and into the back of the throat.
   c. Expose the glottis with the laryngoscope.

Figure 8–1. In a nasotracheal intubation, grasp the tip of the endotracheal tube with Magill forceps and advance the tip below the cords.

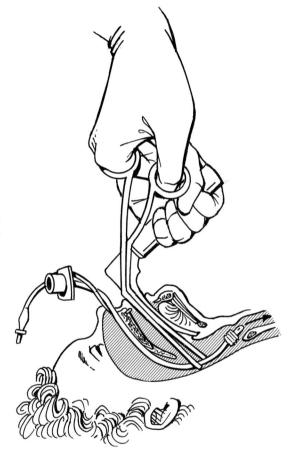

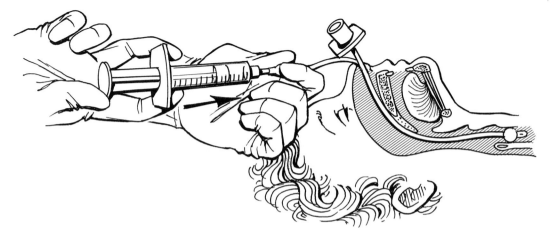

Figure 8–2. Once inserted, gently inflate the cuff with the volume specified on the tube.

    d. An assistant advances the endotracheal tube until the tip is positioned above the cords (it is very difficult for one person to both advance and aim the endotracheal tube).

    e. Grasp the tip of the endotracheal tube with Magill forceps and direct the endotracheal tube between the cords (Fig. 8-1).

    f. Inflate the balloon of the cuffed endotracheal tube (Fig. 8-2).

3. Blind placement

    a. Place the patient in the "sniffing" position.

    b. Insert a lubricated endotracheal tube through the nostril and into the back of the throat.

    c. Listen to the character of the breath sounds transmitted through the endotracheal tube and direct the tube toward the loudest breath sounds. Application of cricoid pressure may shift the airway posteriorly and enhance the chances of intubation of the trachea.

    d. If placement is not successful after a few attempts, the blind route should be abandoned in favor of direct visualization.

COMPLICATIONS

In addition to those complications detailed under oral intubation (see Chapter 7), nasotracheal intubation may be associated with the following:

1. Epistaxis
2. Sinusitis
3. Erosion of the nasal mucosa or septum

References

Black AE, Hatch DJ, Nauth-Misir N. Complication of nasotracheal intubation in neonates, infants, and children: A review of 4 years' experience in a children's hospital. Br J Anaesth 65:461-467, 1990.

Hansen M, Poulsen MR, Bendixen DK, et al. Incidence of sinusitis in patients with nasotracheal intubation. Br J Anaesth 61:231-233, 1988.

CHAPTER 9

Steven Krug

NEEDLE CRICOTHYROIDOTOMY

INDICATIONS

1. A temporary means of ventilation for the patient who cannot be intubated, such as the patient with critical upper airway obstruction because of trauma or an aspirated foreign body.

CONTRAINDICATIONS

None

EQUIPMENT

1. 12- or 14-gauge over-the-needle catheter
2. Syringe: 6- to 12-ml
3. Endotracheal tube adapter: size 3.0
4. Jet ventilation system
   3- to 6-foot high-pressure oxygen tubing
   14 Fr suction catheter, cut to 6 in
   Luer-Lok male connector (A manufactured version is now available commercially.)

PROCEDURE

1. With the patient supine, palpate the cricothyroid membrane between the thyroid and cricoid cartilages (Fig. 9-1).
2. If time permits, prepare the area with Betadine.
3. Attach a 12- or 14-gauge over-the-needle catheter to a 6- to 12-ml syringe.
4. Puncture the skin directly over the cricothyroid membrane at the midline, directing the needle at a 45-degree angle caudally (Fig. 9-2).
5. Insert the needle through the membrane, aspirating as the needle is advanced. Aspiration of air signifies entry into the tracheal lumen.
6. Gently advance the needle downward until it is fully advanced. Some authors recommend withdrawing the stylet and advancing the catheter alone; however, the soft catheter minus the stylet may bend and occlude. Avoid perforation of the posterior wall of the trachea (Fig. 9-2).

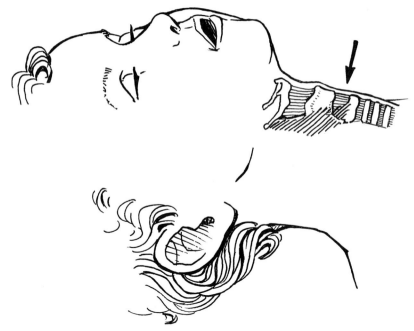

Figure 9–1. Palpate the cricothyroid membrane between the thyroid and cricoid cartilages.

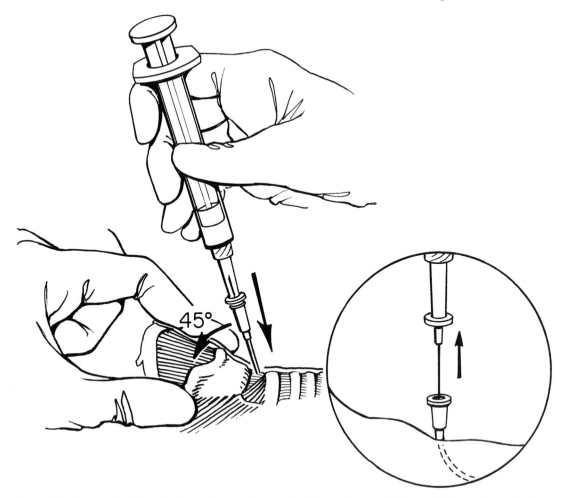

45°

Figure 9–2. Puncture the skin with the needle over the cricothyroid membrane, with the needle directed at a 45-degree angle caudally. Remove the trochar from the angiocath. As the needle enters the trachea, aspirate air to confirm proper position.

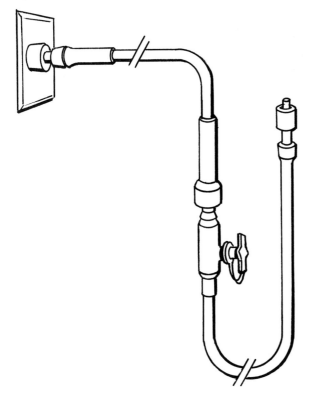

Figure 9–3. Connect the end of the catheter or needle to the Luer-Lok end of jet ventilation system.

7. Connect the catheter or needle stylet hub to the Luer-Lok end of the jet ventilation system (Fig. 9-3). Set the oxygen flow at 15 l/min (30-50 PSI) (Fig. 9-3).
8. Ventilate the patient using a 1:2 ratio (i.e., 1 sec on, 2 sec off). This may be maintained for 30 to 45 min.

COMPLICATIONS

1. Asphyxia
2. Aspiration of blood
3. Exsanguinating hematoma
4. Thyroid perforation
5. Posterior tracheal wall perforation
6. Esophageal perforation
7. Subcutaneous and/or mediastinal emphysema
8. Local infection or cellulitis
9. Inadequate ventilation leading to hypoxia and death

References

Butterworth JF. *Atlas of Procedures in Anesthesia and Critical Care.* Philadelphia, WB Saunders, 1992, pp 37-39.
Chameides L, Hazinski MF (eds). *Textbook of Pediatric Advanced Life Support.* Dallas, American Heart Association, 1994, pp 4-18.
Committee on Trauma. *Advanced Trauma Life Support Course for Physicians.* Chicago, American College of Surgeons, 1989, pp 36-40.
Mace SE: Cricothyrotomy. In Roberts JR, Hedges JR (eds). *Clinical Procedures in Emergency Medicine,* (2nd ed). Philadelphia, WB Saunders, 1991, pp 40-60.
Neff CC, Pfister RC, Van Sonnenberg E. Percutaneous transtracheal ventilation: Experimental and practical aspects. J Trauma 23:84-90, 1983.
Seidman JM. Transtracheal aspiration. In Vander Salm TJ (ed). *Atlas of Bedside Procedures.* Boston, Little, Brown, 1979, pp 151-158.
Stothert JC, Stout MJ, Lewis LM, Keltner RM. High pressure percutaneous transtracheal ventilation: The use of large gauge intravenous-type catheters in the totally obstructed airway. Am J Emerg Med 8:184-189, 1990.

CHAPTER 10

Steven Krug

SURGICAL CRICOTHYROIDOTOMY

INDICATIONS

1. The need for a definitive and secure airway in the patient in whom intubation either by nasal or oral routes is not possible.
2. The need for a secure airway in patients with critical upper airway obstruction above the level of the vocal cords.

CONTRAINDICATIONS

1. Age under 8 yr of age

EQUIPMENT

1. Scalpel
2. Delaborde tracheal spreader or curved hemostat
3. Tracheostomy tube (preferred) or endotracheal tube
4. Pediatric percutaneous tracheostomy kit (Pertrach)

PROCEDURE

1. With the patient in a supine position, palpate the cricothyroid membrane between the cricoid and thyroid cartilages. If possible, slightly hyperextend the neck by placing a rolled towel under the patient's shoulders (see Fig. 9–1).
2. If time permits, prepare the area with Betadine.
3. If the patient is conscious (and if time permits) anesthetize the area with 1% lidocaine.
4. Make an incision into the skin over the lower half of the cricothyroid membrane (Fig. 10–1).
5. Carefully incise through the membrane. The incision must be large enough to permit passage of an appropriate-sized endotracheal or tracheostomy tube.
6. Insert a tracheal spreader or a pair of forceps into the incision and open the airway (Fig. 10–2). An alternate or emergent method would be to insert the scalpel handle through the incision and rotate it 90 degrees to open the airway.

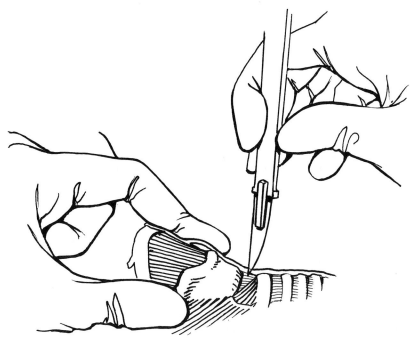

Figure 10–1. Incise the cricothyroid membrane with a scalpel.

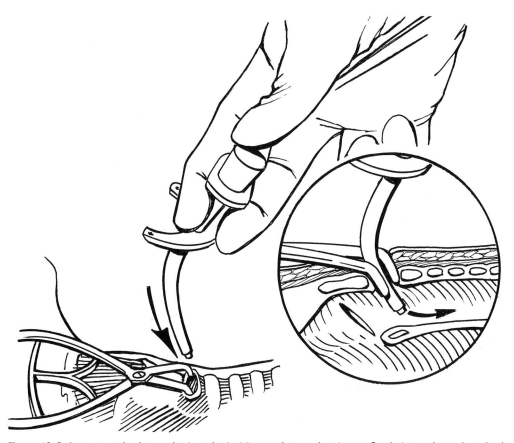

Figure 10–2. Insert a tracheal spreader into the incision, and open the airway. Gently insert the endotracheal tube or tracheostomy tube.

7. Insert an appropriate-sized endotracheal or tracheostomy tube into the incision, directing the tube distally into the tracheal lumen. Inflate the cuff if a cuffed tube is used (Fig. 10-2).
8. Ventilate the patient using an anesthesia or Laerdal bag device, assessing chest rise and breath sounds.
9. Secure the tracheostomy tube in place to prevent its dislodging.

ALTERNATIVE PROCEDURE
(With Pertrach Percutaneous Tracheostomy
Device) (Fig. 10-3)

1-3. Same steps as earlier.
4. Attach the splittable needle from the Pertrach kit to a syringe. Insert the needle through the midpoint of the cricothyroid membrane at a 45-degree caudal angle (Fig. 10-4).
5. As the needle enters the trachea, aspirate air, confirming placement in the tracheal lumen.
6. Carefully remove the syringe while maintaining the position of the needle.
7. Insert the leader of the dilator from the Pertrach device into the needle as far as it will permit (Fig. 10-5).
8. Squeeze the flanges of the needle together and then pull apart the flanges, splitting the needle. It is important to keep the position of the leader wire stable during this procedure.
9. Applying steady pressure, slowly advance the remainder of the leader, the dilator and the tracheostomy tube into the tracheal lumen.
10. Remove the leader and the dilator. Attach the tracheostomy tube to an anesthesia or Laerdal bag device. Confirm placement by the adequacy of ventilation. If correct placement is confirmed, then secure the tube in place with twill tape or tracheostomy ties.

COMPLICATIONS

1. Asphyxia
2. Aspiration of blood
3. Creation of a false passage into the soft tissues of the neck
4. Hemorrhage or hematoma formation
5. Laceration of the trachea
6. Laceration of the esophagus
7. Subcutaneous and/or mediastinal emphysema
8. Vocal cord paralysis
9. Subglottic stenosis or edema
10. Laryngeal stenosis

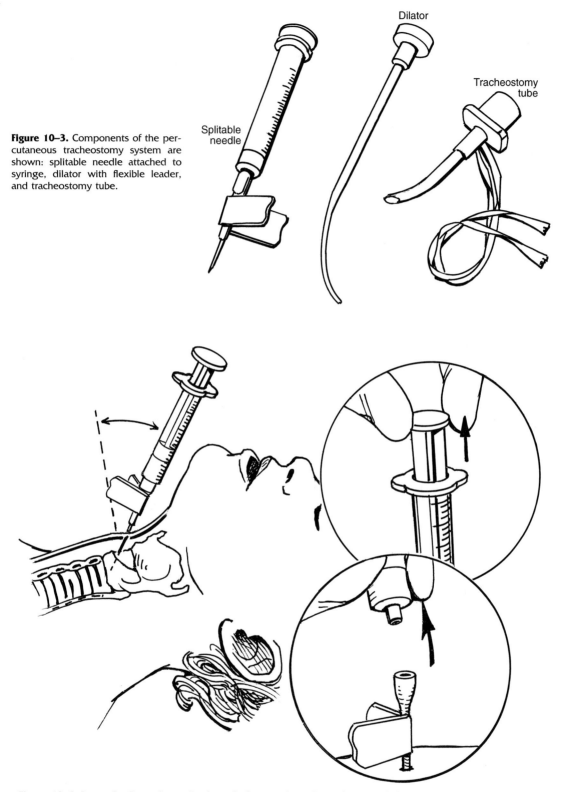

Figure 10–3. Components of the percutaneous tracheostomy system are shown: splitable needle attached to syringe, dilator with flexible leader, and tracheostomy tube.

Dilator

Tracheostomy tube

Splitable needle

Figure 10–4. Insert the Pertrach needle through the cricothyroid membrane and direct the needle at a 45-degree angle caudally. As the needle enters the trachea, aspirate air to confirm proper position. Carefully remove the syringe while maintaining the position of the needle.

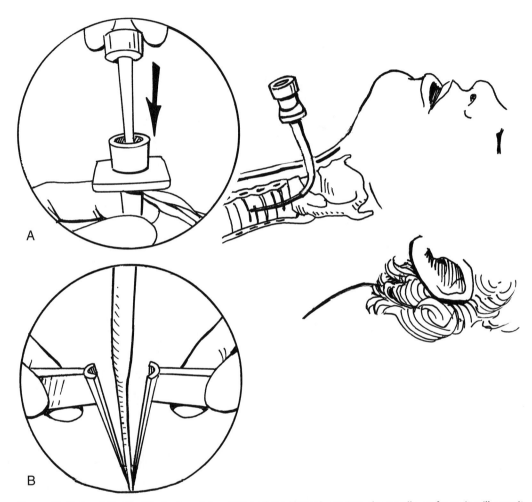

Figure 10–5. Insert the flexible leader of the dilator of the Pertrach set into the needle as far as it will permit (circle A). Thread the flexible leader into the trachea. The needle is then split and removed (circle B). The dilator and tracheostomy tube are together inserted into the trachea.

References

Butterworth JF. *Atlas of Procedures in Anesthesia and Critical Care.* Philadelphia, WB Saunders, 1992, pp 41-44.

Committee on Trauma. *Advanced Trauma Life Support Course for Physicians.* Chicago, American College of Surgeons, 1989, pp 51-55.

Cutler BS. Cricothyroidotomy for emergency airway. In Vander Salm TJ (ed). *Atlas of Bedside Procedures.* Boston, Little, Brown, 1979, pp 169-176.

Mace SE. Cricothyrotomy. In Roberts JR, Hedges JR (eds). *Clinical Procedures in Emergency Medicine* (2nd ed). Philadelphia, WB Saunders, 1991, pp 40-60.

Ruddy RM (ed). Illustrated techniques of pediatric emergency medicine. In Fleisher GR, Ludwig S (eds). *Textbook of Pediatric Emergency Medicine* (3rd ed). Baltimore, Williams and Wilkins, 1993, pp 1620-1621.

Toye FJ, Weinstein JD. Clinical experience with percutaneous tracheostomy and cricothyroidotomy in 100 patients. J Trauma 26:1034-1040, 1986.

CHAPTER 11

Steven Krug

REPLACEMENT OF A TRACHEOSTOMY TUBE

INDICATIONS

1. Accidental decannulation of an existing tracheostomy tube
2. To relieve partial or complete obstruction of a tracheostomy tube because of a foreign body, mucus plug, or excessive secretions

CONTRAINDICATIONS

Inadequate available equipment (e.g., a replacement tube)

EQUIPMENT

1. Anesthesia or Laerdal bag and mask
2. Suction catheter
3. Replacement tracheostomy tube (same size or one size smaller); (if these are not available, then an age-appropriate–sized endotracheal tube may be substituted)
4. Scissors
5. Oxygen catheter, 10 or 14 Fr
6. Tracheostomy ties or twill tape

PROCEDURE FOR THE MANAGEMENT AND/OR REPLACEMENT OF AN OBSTRUCTED TUBE

1. If respiratory distress is present, attempt to ventilate the child through the tracheostomy tube with 100% oxygen using an anesthesia or Laerdal bag.
2. If this is not successful, attempt to pass a suction catheter through the tracheostomy tube. If the catheter passes, provide suction (80–100 cm of water) for 3 to 5 sec, then reattempt ventilation through the tracheostomy tube.
3. If it remains impossible to ventilate the patient through the tube, then the tube will require replacement. Remember to consider ventilating the patient "from above," using a bag and mask.
4. Before removing the present tracheostomy tube, locate and prepare a new tube for placement. This preparation should include attaching an adequate length of twill tape to the flange of the tube to allow for proper securing around the

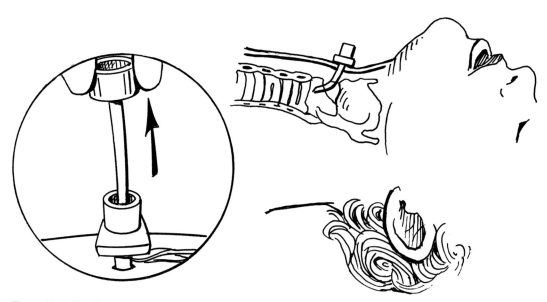

Figure 11–1. The dilator is removed, leaving the tracheostomy tube in place.

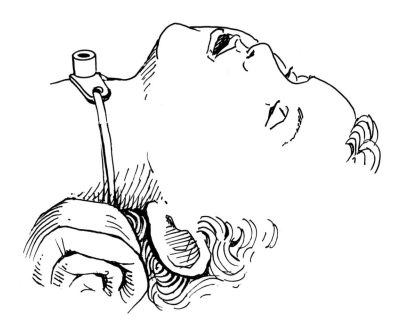

Figure 11–2. Extend the patient's neck, cut the tracheostomy ties, and remove the old trach.

patient's neck. If a new tube is not available, an endotracheal tube may be used on a temporary basis. If an endotracheal tube is used, it should not be advanced beyond the carina (the tube can be shorted by removing the adapter, cutting the proximal end of the tube to a length midway between that of the tracheostomy tube and the estimated distance from the stoma to the carina, and then replacing the adapter). In an emergency, the original tracheostomy tube can be reused, providing its lumen and tip are cleared of obstructive materials.

5. Extend the patient's neck by placing a towel beneath the child's shoulders. If they are present, cut the tracheostomy ties and remove the tube.

6. Insert a new tube (with the dilator tip in place) into the tracheostomy stoma. This should pass easily, and excessive force should not be required. Confirm placement of the tube by removing the dilator and ventilating the patient with an anesthesia or Laerdal bag (Fig. 11-1).

7. If one is unable to insert the tube, or if excessive force is required (do not force the tube in place, as it may result in the creation of a false tracheal passage!), follow the procedure for the replacement of a dislodged tube. Also consider the insertion of a tracheostomy tube one size smaller than the original, or as described above, an appropriate-sized endotracheal tube.

PROCEDURE FOR THE REPLACEMENT OF A DISLODGED TUBE

1. If respiratory distress is present, attempt to ventilate the patient "from above" using a bag and mask and 100% oxygen. Remember to occlude the stoma site with a finger when performing bag-mask ventilation.

2. As time may not permit the location and preparation of a replacement tracheostomy tube, one should consider replacing the dislodged tube (if present), or using an appropriate-sized endotracheal tube as a temporizing procedure.

3. Extend the patient's neck by placing a towel beneath the child's shoulders. If present, cut the tracheostomy ties and remove the tube.

4. If time permits (or after the placement of an endotracheal tube), prepare a tracheostomy tube as described earlier.

5. Attempt placement of the tracheostomy tube with its dilator in place as described earlier. If this is difficult or unsuccessful, pass an oxygen catheter (with an oxygen flow rate of 1 to 2 l/min) into the tracheostomy stoma. The catheter will serve as a guide for the tracheostomy tube (Fig. 11-2).

6. Cut the oxygen catheter with scissors, leaving a length approximately twice the distance from the stoma to the carina.

7. Remove the tracheostomy dilator and pass the tube over the catheter into the stoma. If this proves difficult, consider using a tube one size smaller than the patient's original (Fig. 11-3). If the tube passes easily, the catheter should be removed and airway patency established.

COMPLICATIONS

1. Respiratory distress or failure
2. Creation of a false tracheal passage

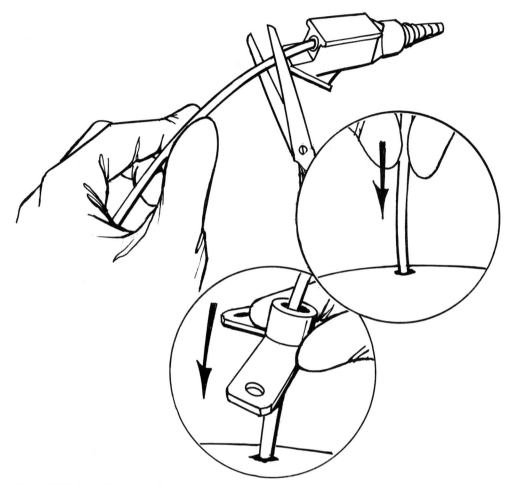

Figure 11–3. A small-gauge catheter may be used as a guide when replacing a tracheostomy tube. Cut off any connecting apparatus from the catheter, leaving a length that is twice the distance from the stoma to the carina. Slide the catheter into the old tracheostomy tube, remove the old tube, and slide the new tracheostomy tube into the trachea. The same technique can be used if the trach has become dislodged and the stoma is difficult to recannulate.

3. Pneumomediastinum
4. Pneumothorax
5. Hemorrhage

References

Chameides L, Hazinski MF (eds). *Textbook of Pediatric Advanced Life Support.* Dallas, American Heart Association, pp 4-20, 4-21, 1994.

Ruddy RM (ed). Illustrated Techniques of Pediatric Emergency Medicine. In Fleisher GR, Ludwig S (eds). *Textbook of Pediatric Emergency Medicine,* (3rd ed). Baltimore, Williams and Wilkins, pp 1622-1623, 1993.

SECTION 3

VASCULAR ACCESS

CHAPTER 12

Michele Walsh-Sukys

PERIPHERAL AND SCALP INTRAVENOUS CATHETER

INDICATIONS

1. Administration of medications
2. Administration of fluids and/or parenteral nutrition to patients in whom enteral feeding is undesirable

CONTRAINDICATIONS

None

EQUIPMENT

1. Gloves
2. Tourniquet or rubber band
3. Alcohol wipes
4. T connector
5. Saline or heparinized saline flush
6. Angiocaths in sizes appropriate to neonate or child
7. Tape
8. Sterile 2 × 2
9. Band-Aid
10. Armboards
11. Gauze rolls or other stabilizing materials

TECHNIQUE

1. Obtain supplemental light and heating lamps as needed.
2. Wash hands thoroughly.
3. Attach syringe of flush solution to T connector and flush through.
4. Examine extremities (and scalp in infants) for the best site (Figs. 12–1, 12–2,

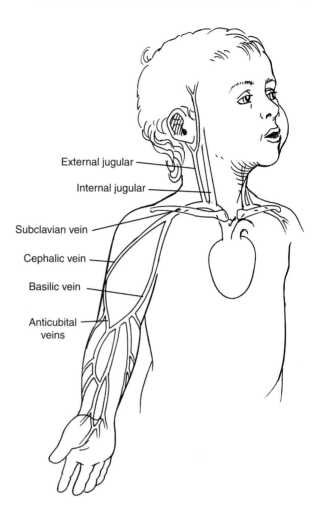

Figure 12–1. Venous anatomy of the arm and neck. The most commonly used sites are the cephalic and basilic veins.

External jugular

Internal jugular

Subclavian vein

Cephalic vein

Basilic vein

Anticubital veins

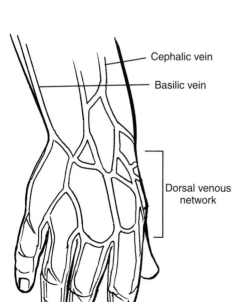

Cephalic vein

Basilic vein

Dorsal venous network

Figure 12–2. Venous anatomy of the dorsum of the hand. Because of their visible and superficial location, the veins of the hand are the preferred venous site.

12-3). It is wise to begin at the most distal sites and work proximally if attempts are unsuccessful.

5. Apply tourniquet (or rubber band in a neonate).
6. Put on gloves.
7. Cleanse 2-cm area surrounding site with alcohol allowing at least 30 sec to dry.
8. Immobilize insertion site with nondominant hand.
9. Hold the angiocath at a 30-degree angle with the bevel up, and puncture insertion site superficially a few millimeters distal to the point at which you wish to enter the vein.
10. Gently advance the catheter with the stylet in place until the vessel is entered. You may feel a "pop" when the vessel is entered, and with most larger catheters you should get a blood return into the catheter hub (Fig. 12-4).
11. If no blood return is obtained, you may check for correct placement by removing the stylet and flushing with 0.5 to 2 ml of fluid.
12. If flushing reveals infiltration, remove catheter and hold pressure with sterile gauze.
13. If an artery is inadvertently entered, hold pressure for a minimum of 3 min.
14. If the catheter is successfully placed, gently advance the catheter until the hub is adjacent to the skin.
15. Secure catheter, T connector, and syringe with tape or transparent dressing.
16. In pediatrics it is imperative to protect the angiocath from curious hands and mouths by covering the angiocath with a protective dressing such as an inverted medicine cup or gauze rolls. It is usually best to immobilize the extremity on an intravenous injection (IV) board appropriate to size. Label all sites with the date and time of placement and the size of the catheter.

COMPLICATIONS

1. Intra-arterial insertion or laceration of adjacent artery.
2. Infection: Failure to use aseptic technique may lead to phlebitis or bacteremia.
3. Infiltration: Hyperosmolar or irritating substances may cause damage to surrounding tissues. Infiltration of calcium-containing fluids or inotropic agents may be especially destructive.
   a. Elevating the extremity and wrapping the extremity in a warm compress may speed reabsorption of the infiltrate.
   b. Topical application of 2% nitroglycerin paste (no more than 4 mm/kg) has also been shown to be helpful. If infiltrates are extensive enough to cause blistering, surgical consultation should be obtained.
   c. Injection of hyaluronidase at the site of IV infiltrate may speed resorption of the infiltrated fluid and therefore limit secondary injury owing to local capillary compromise.

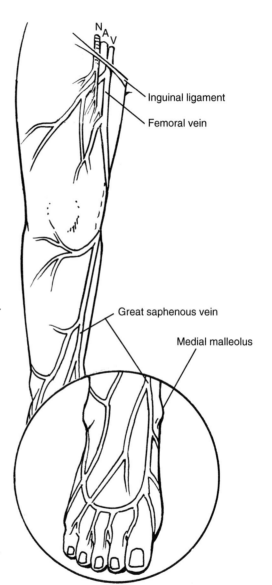

Figure 12–3. Venous anatomy of the foot and leg.

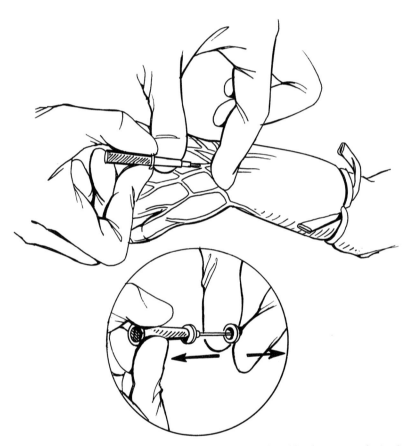

Figure 12–4. Puncture the vessel with the angiocath. When blood return is obtained, advance the catheter while simultaneously withdrawing the stylet.

References

Batton DG, Maisels MJ, Applebaum P. Use of peripheral intravenous cannulas in premature infants: A controlled study. Pediatrics 70:487, 1982.

Flanigan DP, Keifer TJ, Schuler JJ, et al. Experience with iatrogenic pediatric vascular injuries. Ann Surg 198:430, 1983.

Raszka WV, Kueser TK, Smith FR, Bass JW. The use of hyaluronidase in the treatment of intravenous extravasation injuries. J Perinatol 10:146–150, 1990.

Wong AF, McCulloch LM, Sola A. Treatment of peripheral tissue ischemia with topical nitroglycerin ointment in neonates. J Pediatr 121:980, 1992.

CHAPTER 13

Michele Walsh-Sukys

PERIPHERAL PERCUTANEOUS ARTERIAL CATHETER PLACEMENT

INDICATIONS

1. Continuous monitoring of arterial pressure
2. Need for frequent arterial blood samples

CONTRAINDICATIONS

1. Absent collateral arterial supply

EQUIPMENT

1. Gloves
2. Tourniquet or rubber band
3. Alcohol wipes
4. T connector
5. Saline or heparinized saline flush
6. Angiocaths in sizes appropriate to neonate or child
7. Tape
8. Sterile 2 × 2
9. Band-Aid
10. Armboards
11. Gauze rolls or other stabilizing materials

TECHNIQUE

1. Obtain supplemental light and heating lamps as needed.
2. Wash hands thoroughly.
3. Attach syringe of flush solution to T connector and flush through.
4. Examine extremities for the best site. The most widely used sites are the radial, dorsalis pedis, and posterior tibial arteries. Confirm presence of collateral circulation. If using the radial artery, this can be performed using the Allen test (Fig. 13-1). Occlude both the radial and ulnar arteries *(A)*. The patient then

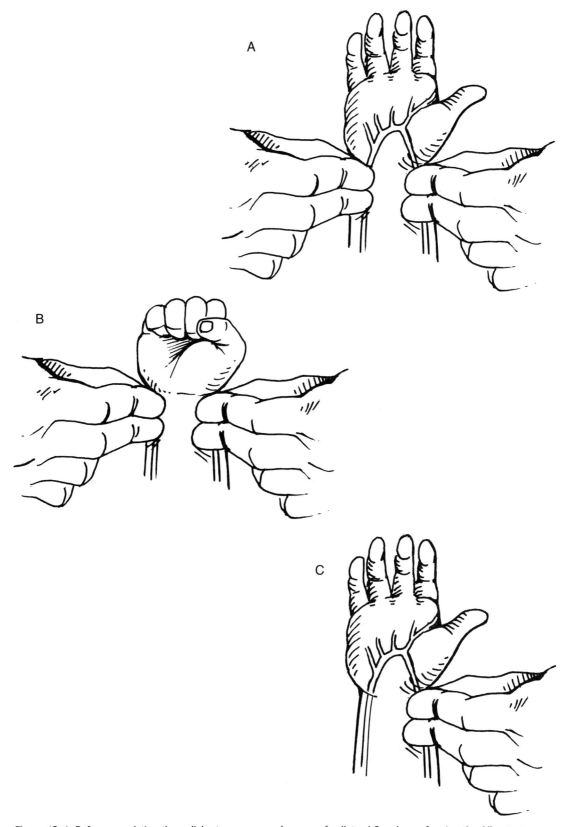

Figure 13–1. Before cannulating the radial artery, ensure adequacy of collateral flow by performing the Allen test.

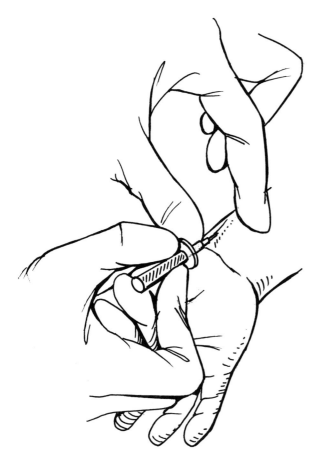

Figure 13–2. Palpate the artery with the nondominant hand and gently advance the catheter at a 30- to 45-degree angle until the artery is entered.

squeezes the hand until the hand is pale *(B)*. If the patient is unable to cooperate, the hand may be squeezed by the examiner. Release the pressure on the ulnar artery, and observe for rapid (less than 5 sec) refill of blood *(C)*. If this does not occur, collateral circulation is inadequate and the radial artery should not be used.

5. Put on gloves.
6. Cleanse 2-cm area surrounding site with alcohol, allowing at least 30 sec to dry.
7. Palpate arterial pulse with nondominant hand. Gently hyperextend the joint to decrease the motion of the artery.
8. Hold the angiocath at a 30-degree angle with the bevel up and puncture insertion site superficially a few millimeters away from the point where you wish to enter the artery (Fig. 13–2).
9. Gently advance the catheter with the stylet in place until the artery is entered. You may feel a "pop" when the artery is entered.
10. Remove the stylet and confirm arterial flow.
11. Advance the catheter with a gentle "screwing" motion.
12. Secure catheter, T-connector, and syringe with tape or transparent dressing.

COMPLICATIONS

1. Laceration of artery
2. Necrosis of distal sites owing to loss of arterial flow distal to the catheter, related to hematoma, arteriospasm, or thrombosis. Adequate collateral circulation must be ensured before catheter placement by occluding the artery and confirming that blanching does not occur.
3. Infection: Failure to use aseptic technique may lead to phlebitis or bacteremia. Osteomyelitis has been described. Infection of the hip joint can be particularly associated with femoral puncture.
4. Embolization: Air or particulate debris can be embolized to distal capillary beds, causing local infarction. Meticulous catheter care can minimize this complication.
5. Nerve injury: Particularly vulnerable sites include median nerve (brachial artery), posterior tibial nerve (posterior tibial artery), and femoral nerve (femoral artery).
6. Hemorrhage

References

Goetzman BW. Arterial access in the newborn. Am J Dis Child 141:841, 1987.
Randel SN, Tsang BH, Wung JT, et al. Experience with percutaneous indwelling peripheral arterial catheterization in neonates. Am J Dis Child 141:848, 1987.
Shaw JC. Arterial blood sampling from the radial artery in premature and full term infants. Lancet 2:389, 1968.

CHAPTER 14

Michele Walsh-Sukys

PERCUTANEOUS FEMORAL VENOUS CATHETERIZATION

INDICATIONS

1. Lack of peripheral venous cannulation sites
2. Administration of medications that irritate venous tissue
3. Need to simultaneously infuse multiple incompatible medications through multiple lumens
4. Delivery of parenteral nutrition containing >12.5% dextrose solution
5. Need for central venous access for hemodynamic monitoring or for transvenous cardiac pacing

CONTRAINDICATIONS

1. Skin infection overlying site
2. Relative contraindications:
   Bleeding diathesis that is uncontrolled
   Obese patient

EQUIPMENT

1. Sterile gloves, gowns, masks, drapes
2. Betadine solution
3. Alcohol wipes
4. T connector
5. Saline or heparinized saline flush
6. Single-, double-, or triple-lumen venous catheter appropriate to patient size
7. Tape
8. Sterile gauze sponges
9. 18- or 20-gauge needle or angiocath; syringe
10. 50-cm guidewire small enough to pass easily through introduced needle (0.035 inch is typically adequate)
11. Scalpel (#11)
12. Dilator
13. Radiopaque catheter of length appropriate to patient

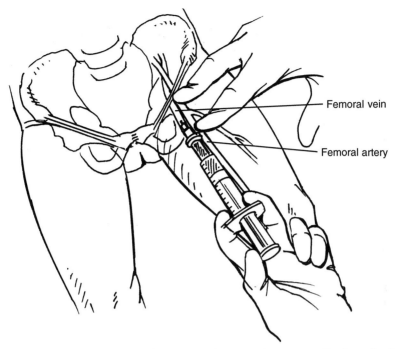

— Femoral vein

— Femoral artery

Figure 14–1. Knowledge of the anatomy of the femoral triangle is crucial to success. The femoral vein lies 4 to 6 mm medial to the femoral artery at the base of the inguinal ligament. The mnemonic NAVY will aid memory: (from lateral to medial), nerve, artery, vein, Y (representing the junction of the legs).

Figure 14–2. The Seldinger technique is used to place the femoral venous line. Catheterize the vein with the introducer needle.

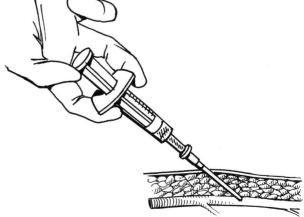
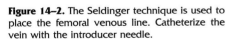

TECHNIQUE

1. Obtain supplemental light and heating lamps as needed. Place roll under hip on selected side to elevate the femoral triangle. Keep knee extended and foot rotated externally by 15 to 30 degrees.
2. Wash hands thoroughly.
3. Cleanse wide area surrounding site with alcohol or Betadine, allowing at least 30 sec for solution to dry.
4. Put on sterile mask, gown, and glove. Cover the area with sterile drapes.
5. Attach syringe of flush solution to T connector and flush through. If inserting a multiple-lumen catheter, flush all ports and lumens.
6. Infiltrate the area with a 25-gauge needle and syringe with 1% lidocaine without epinephrine.
7. Identify femoral triangle (Fig. 14-1). Palpate arterial pulse with nondominant hand just below the inguinal ligament. The vein is located 4 to 6 mm medial to the femoral pulse.
8. Hold the needle at a 30- to 45-degree angle with the bevel up, and puncture insertion site two fingerwidths below the inguinal ligament or inguinal skinfold.
9. Gently advance the needle until the vein is entered and flashback of venous blood is confirmed. You may feel a "pop" when the vessel is entered (Fig. 14-2). Remove the syringe and occlude the hub to prevent air embolism.
10. Place the guidewire through the needle, ensuring it reaches beyond the tip of the needle into the iliac vein (Fig. 14-3). The guidewire should advance easily without resistance. It should never be forced. An assistant should always hold the distal end of the guidewire to ensure against migration into or out of the vessel.
11. Remove the introducer needle. Make a nick in the skin with the scalpel at the wire, take care not to cut the wire. The dilator is then advanced with a twisting motion through the skin and subcutaneous tissue. Remove the dilator (Fig. 14-4).
12. Thread the catheter over the wire (Fig. 14-5). When the catheter is in place, stabilize the catheter against the skin and withdraw the wire. Attach T connector and syringe. In turn, aspirate venous blood and then flush all catheter ports.
13. Secure catheter, T connector, and syringe with a suture, and then cover with a sterile dressing.

COMPLICATIONS

1. Arterial puncture
2. Venous thrombosis with possible pulmonary emboli
3. Arrythmias
4. Infection: Failure to use aseptic technique, leading to phlebitis or bacteremia
5. Embolization: By air or particulate debris (meticulous catheter care can minimize this complication)
6. Femoral nerve injury

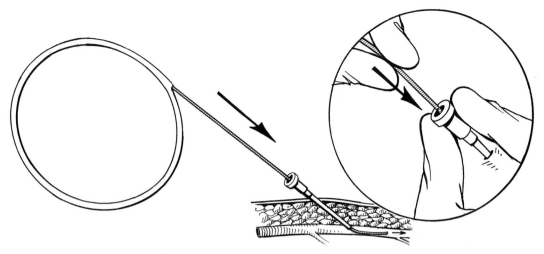

Figure 14–3. Advance the guidewire through the introducer needle while ensuring that the introducer needle is stabilized. The guidewire should advance easily without resistance.

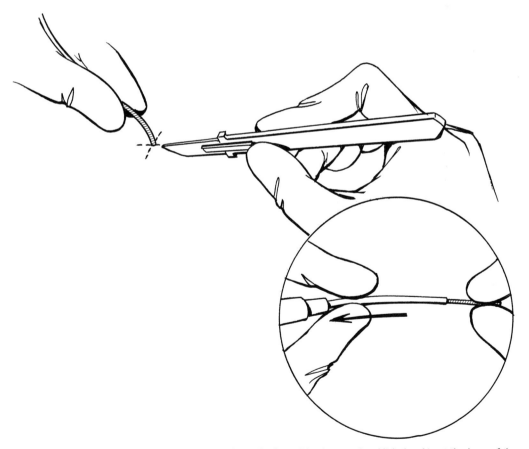

Figure 14–4. After removing the introducer needle, only the guidewire remains. Nick the skin at the base of the guidewire to enlarge the opening and advance the dilator over the wire.

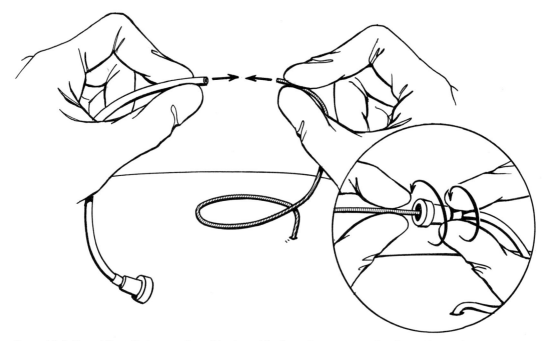

Figure 14–5. Thread the catheter over the guidewire, while the assistant ensures that the guidewire does not migrate. Withdraw the guidewire.

References

Kanter RK, Gorton JM, Palmiere K, et al. Anatomy of femoral vessels in infants and guidelines for venous catheterization. Pediatrics 83:1020-1024, 1989.

Kanter RK, Zimmerman JJ, Strauss RH, Stoeckel KA. Central venous catheter insertion by femoral vein: Safety and effectiveness for pediatric patients. Pediatrics 77:842-845, 1986.

Seldinger SI. Catheter replacement of the needle in percutaneous arteriography: A new technique. Acta Radiol Diagn 39:368-371, 1953.

Stenzel JP, Green TP, Fuhrman BP, et al. Percutaneous femoral venous catheterizations: A prospective study of complications. J Pediatr 114:411-415, 1989.

Swanson RS, Uhlig PN, Gross PL, et al. Emergency intravenous access through the femoral vein. Ann Emerg Med 13:244-248, 1984.

CHAPTER 15

Michele Walsh-Sukys

PERCUTANEOUS FEMORAL ARTERIAL CATHETERIZATION

INDICATIONS

1. Continuous monitoring of arterial pressure
2. Need for frequent arterial blood samples

CONTRAINDICATIONS

1. Coagulation abnormality
2. Skin infection overlying site

EQUIPMENT

1. Gloves
2. Betadine solution
3. Alcohol wipes
4. T connector
5. Saline or heparinized saline flush
6. Single-lumen arterial catheter
7. Tape
8. Sterile 2 × 2
9. Band-Aid

TECHNIQUE

1. Obtain supplemental light and heating lamps as needed. Place roll under hip on selected side to elevate the femoral triangle.
2. Wash hands thoroughly.
3. Attach syringe of flush solution to T connector and flush through.
4. Cleanse 2-cm area surrounding site with alcohol or Betadine, allowing at least 30 sec for solution to dry.
5. Put on sterile gloves. Cover the area with sterile drapes.
6. Infiltrate the area with a 25-gauge needle and syringe with 1% lidocaine without epinephrine.
7. Identify femoral triangle (Fig. 15–1). Palpate arterial pulse with nondominant hand just below the inguinal ligament.
8. Hold the needle at a 30- to 45-degree angle with the bevel up, and puncture insertion site two fingerwidths below the inguinal ligament or inguinal skinfold.
9. Gently advance the needle until the artery is entered and flashback of arterial

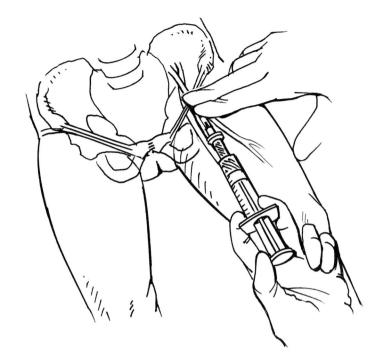

Figure 15–1. Identify the femoral artery by palpation at the base of the inguinal ligament. Introduce the needle slowly while continuously aspirating on the syringe.

blood is confirmed. You may feel a "pop" when the artery is entered. (See also Figs. 14-3, 14-5.)

10. Place the guidewire through the needle, ensuring it reaches beyond the tip of the needle. Remove the needle, and thread the catheter over the wire.

11. Secure catheter, T connector, and syringe with tape or transparent dressing.

12. Assess patency once again by observing pressure wave form and free-flowing blood return. Immediately assess perfusion distal to the catheter and ensure that adequate flow is present. Document adequacy of flow in the procedure note.

COMPLICATIONS

1. Laceration of artery
2. Necrosis of distal sites owing to loss of arterial flow distal to the catheter related to hematoma, arteriospasm, or thrombosis
3. Infection: Failure to use aseptic technique may lead to phlebitis or bacteremia. Osteomyelitis of the femoral head or septic arthritis has been described and is a particular risk in neonates.
4. Embolization: Air or particulate debris can be embolized to distal capillary beds, causing local infarction. Meticulous catheter care can minimize this complication.
5. Femoral nerve injury

References

Fleming R, Friedman S. Late sequelae after femoral artery catheterization. Am J Cardiol 53:1205-1209, 1984.

Gurman GM, Kriemerman S. Cannulation of big arteries in critically ill patients. Crit Care Med 13:217-222, 1985.

Purdue GF, Hunt JL. Vascular access through the femoral vessels: Indications and complications. J Burn Care Rehabil 7:498-452, 1986.

Puri VK, Carlson RC, Bander JJ, et al. Complications of vascular catheterization in the critically ill. Crit Care Med 8:495-499, 1991.

Thomas F, Burke JP, Parker J, et al. The risk of infection related to radial vs femoral sites for arterial catheterization. Crit Care Med 11:807-811, 1983.

CHAPTER 16

James R. Harley

EXTERNAL JUGULAR VENOUS CANNULATION

INDICATIONS

1. Vascular access when other peripheral veins cannot be cannulated
2. Central venous pressure (CVP) (when a long catheter is placed with Seldinger's technique)

CONTRAINDICATIONS

1. Patients with suspected cervical spine injury
2. Patients with respiratory distress or partial airway obstruction, as they may not tolerate positioning for the procedure

EQUIPMENT

1. IV catheter (18- to 22-gauge)
2. IV tubing
3. IV fluid
4. Tape
5. Towel roll
6. Betadine
7. Central line kit if Seldinger's technique is used (introducer needle, 1% lidocaine, 22- and 27-gauge needles, 5- and 10-cc syringes, guidewire, dilator, catheter, scalpel, suture, Betadine solution, sterile towels, and heparin flush 100 U/cc of normal saline)

PROCEDURE FOR CATHETER INSERTION

1. Place the patient in a supine position with a towel roll under the shoulders. Tilt the bed to a Trendelenburg position of 30 degrees (Fig. 16-1).
2. Restrain the child and have an assistant hold the head by the forehead or chin. The head should be turned away from the side to be punctured (provided the cervical spine has been cleared of possible injury).
3. Identify the external jugular vein. Place gentle pressure on the vein proximal to the site to be entered to distend the vessel (Fig. 16-2).

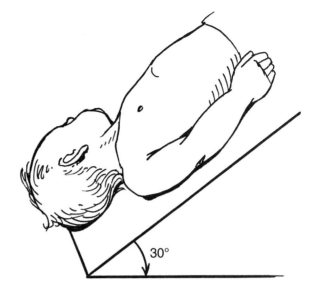

Figure 16–1. Position the patient supine, and in the Trendelenburg position.

30°

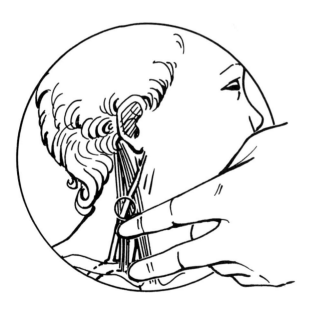

Figure 16–2. Identify the external jugular vein where it crosses the sternocleidomastoid muscle and apply gentle pressure proximal to the site to distend the vessel.

4. Prepare the site with Betadine solution.
5. Enter the skin with the catheter attached to a syringe at a point one half to two thirds of the distance from the angle of the jaw and the clavicle. Keep traction and pressure on the skin over the vein. Gently aspirate the syringe while slowly advancing the needle toward the vein (Fig. 16–3).
6. Once blood is obtained, advance the catheter another 1 to 2 mm (without withdrawing the stylet) until the catheter tip is completely inside the vein. Withdraw the stylet 1 to 2 mm and advance the catheter to the hub; then remove the stylet.
7. Connect to IV tubing.
8. Secure the catheter to the skin with tape or suture.

ALTERNATIVE PROCEDURE: SELDINGER'S TECHNIQUE FOR CVP PLACEMENT
(See Chapter 14 Femoral Venous Catheterization.)

1. Same as steps 1 through 5 above.
6. Estimate the length of catheter insertion by measuring the distance from the catheter site to the junction of the manubrium and sternum.
7. Flush the CVP catheter ports with heparin flush (100 U/cc).
8. Consider local infiltration with lidocaine for local anesthesia.
9. Enter the external jugular with an introducer needle attached to a syringe. Insertion site should be at a point one half to two thirds of the distance from the angle of the jaw to the clavicle.
10. Keep traction and gentle pressure on the skin over the vein proximally.
11. When blood is obtained, stabilize the needle with one hand and remove the syringe with the other.
12. Cover the end of the needle with a gloved finger.
13. Advance a flexible J-wire through the needle.
14. Remove the needle, while holding the guidewire in place. Take care not to cut the wire.
15. Make a small nick in the skin with a scalpel where the guidewire enters the skin.
16. Advance the catheter over the wire the predetermined length. Never let go of the guidewire.
17. Remove the guidewire.
18. Aspirate blood with a syringe to confirm placement and then flush with heparin solution.
19. Connect the catheter to IV tubing.
20. Secure the catheter to the skin with tape or sutures.
21. Confirm placement with an x-ray examination.

COMPLICATIONS

1. Infection
2. Pneumothorax
3. Pneumomediastinum
4. Hematoma
5. Hemothorax
6. Chylothorax

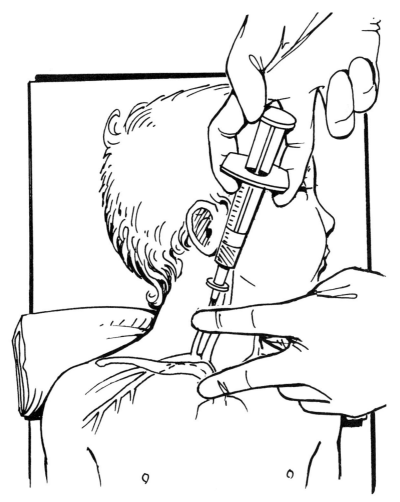

Figure 16–3. Enter the vessel at a measured distance, which is equal to one half to two thirds the distance from the angle of the jaw to the clavicle.

7. Dysrhythmia (Seldinger)
8. Air embolus
9. Catheter or wire (Seldinger) embolus
10. Thrombosis

References

Barker WJ. Central venous catheterization: Internal jugular approach and alternatives. In Roberts JR, Hedges JR (eds). *Clinical Procedures in Emergency Medicine* (2nd ed). Philadelphia, WB Saunders, 1991, pp 345-346.

Carlson DW, Digiulio GA, Gewitz MH, et al. Illustrated techniques of pediatric emergency procedures. In Fleisher GR, Ludwig S (eds). *Textbook of Pediatric Emergency Medicine* (3rd ed). Baltimore, Williams and Wilkins, 1993, pp 1576-1577.

Chameides L. *Textbook of Pediatric Advanced Life Support.* Dallas, American Heart Association, 1988, pp 39-41.

CHAPTER 17

Jim R. Harley

INTERNAL JUGULAR VENOUS CANNULATION

INDICATIONS

1. Central IV access
2. Central venous pressure (CVP) measurement
3. Insertion of Swan-Ganz catheter

CONTRAINDICATIONS

1. Potential C-spine injury
2. Bleeding diathesis

EQUIPMENT

1. Towel roll
2. Tape
3. Central line catheter kit (introducer needle, 1% lidocaine, 22- and 27-gauge needles, 5- and 10-cc syringes, guidewire, dilator, catheter, scalpel, suture, Betadine solution, sterile towels, and heparin flush 100 U/cc of normal saline)

PROCEDURE

1. Place the child in Trendelenburg position of 20 to 30 degrees. Insert a towel roll under the shoulders. The patient's head should be turned slightly away from the side of venipuncture. The right side is preferred (see Fig. 16–1).
2. Place the child on a cardiac monitor.
3. Identify the insertion point, using one of the three following approaches:
   Medial or Central Approach (Figs. 17–1 and 17–2). Find the needle insertion point at the apex of the triangle formed by the sternal and clavicular heads of the sternocleidomastoid muscle. The skin is punctured at the identified insertion point. Direct the needle caudally and laterally at a 45- to 60°-angle to the coronal plane toward the ipsilateral nipple. The path of needle insertion

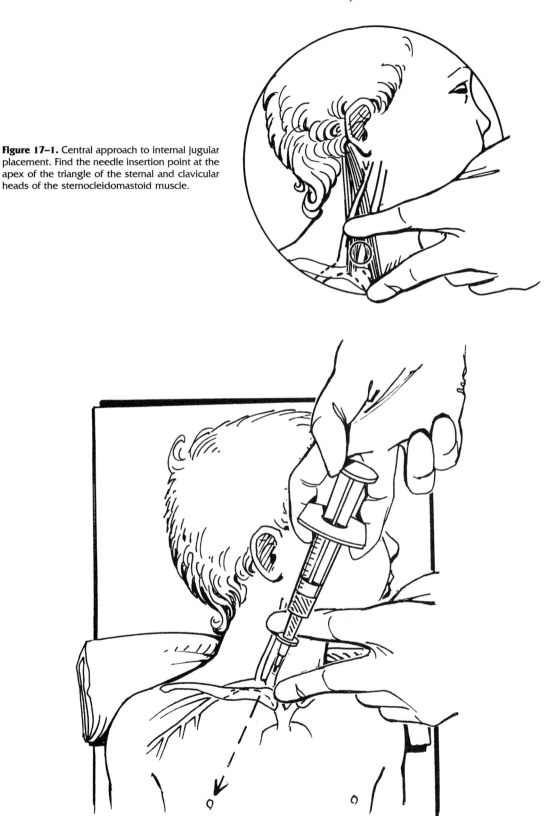

Figure 17–1. Central approach to internal jugular placement. Find the needle insertion point at the apex of the triangle of the sternal and clavicular heads of the sternocleidomastoid muscle.

Figure 17–2. Central approach to internal jugular placement. Direct the needle caudally and laterally toward the ipsilateral nipple. The path should be parallel to the medial border of the clavicular head of the sternocleidomastoid.

should be parallel to the medial border of the clavicular head of the sternoclei-domastoid.

Anterior Approach (Fig. 17-3). The needle insertion site is at the mid-point of the medial edge of the sternocleidomastoid muscle. The needle is then directed toward the ipsilateral nipple down at an angle of 30 to 45 degrees to the coronal plane.

Posterior Approach (Figs. 17-4 and 17-5). The needle is inserted at the lateral margin of the junction of the lower and middle third of the sternocleido-mastoid muscle. The needle is then directed caudally and medially toward the sternal notch under the sternocleidomastoid muscle.

4. Estimate the length of catheter insertion by measuring the distance from the insertion site to the manubrium-sternal junction (see also Chapter 14).
5. Prepare the site with Betadine and cover the area with sterile towels.
6. Anesthetize the area of insertion with 1% lidocaine.
7. The vein can be located with either the introducer needle attached to a syringe or a small "locator needle" (tuberculin syringe and needle). By using a small-gauge needle such as on a tuberculin syringe, one can determine the location of the internal jugular vein then use the introducer needle. This technique helps minimize accidental carotid puncture.
8. As the needle is advanced, negative pressure should always be applied to the syringe when the needle is advanced or retracted.
9. When venous blood is aspirated, the syringe is removed. The hub of the needle should be covered immediately with a thumb to prevent an air embolus during inspiration.
10. The guidewire is then introduced. The guidewire should advance easily without force. If a rhythm change is seen, withdraw the guidewire 1 cm. If the guidewire does not advance easily, remove it, relocate the vein with the introducer needle, and reinsert the guidewire. If the guidewire meets resistance on removal, do not apply excessive force but remove the introducer needle and wire together, check the guidewire to see if it needs replacing, then reinsert the introducer needle.
11. Remove the introducer needle. Stabilize the guidewire. Never let go of the guidewire until it is removed from the patient.
12. Make a small nick in the skin over the guidewire to facilitate catheter entry. Take care not to cut the wire (see Fig. 14-4).
13. Insert the dilator over the guidewire (see Fig. 14-5).
14. Remove the dilator.
15. Insert the catheter over the guidewire. Placement should be at the junction of the right atrium and superior vena cava.
16. Aspirate blood to confirm placement.
17. Connect port to intravenous (IV) tubing. Flush unconnected ports with heparin flush.
18. Obtain an x-ray examination to confirm proper placement.
19. Secure catheter to skin with sutures.

COMPLICATIONS

1. Pneumothorax
2. Pneumomediastinum
3. Hemothorax

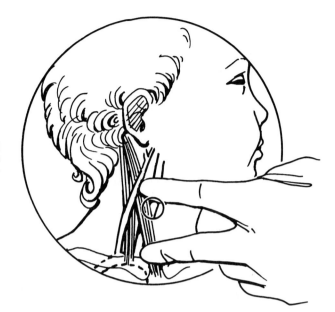

Figure 17–3. Anterior approach to internal jugular placement. The needle insertion point is at the middle of the medial sternocleidomastoid muscle.

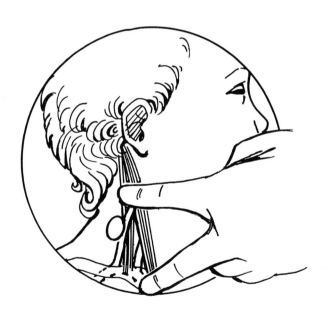

Figure 17–4. Posterior approach to internal jugular placement. The needle insertion point is at the lateral margin of the junction of the lower and middle third of the sternocleidomastoid muscle.

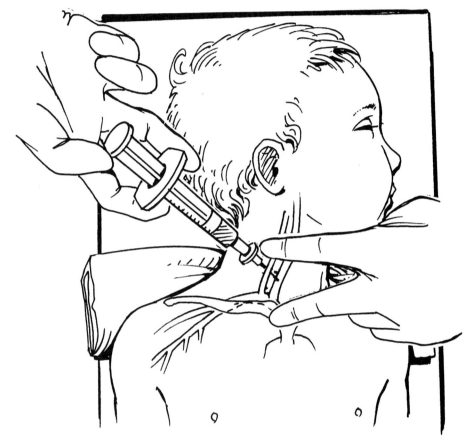

Figure 17–5. Posterior approach to internal jugular placement. The needle is inserted underneath the *external* jugular vein and then enters the *internal* jugular vein.

4. Hydrothorax
5. Chylothorax
6. Dysrhythmia
7. Air embolus
8. Catheter embolus
9. Hematoma (bilateral hematomas may obstruct airway)
10. Local infection
11. Bacteremia/sepsis
12. Thrombosis

References

Barker WJ. Central venous catheterization: Internal jugular approach and alternatives. In Roberts JR, Hedges JR (eds). *Clinical Procedures in Emergency Medicine* (2nd ed). Philadelphia, WB Saunders, 1991, pp 284-287.

Carlson DW, Digiulio GA, Gewitz MH, et al. Illustrated techniques of pediatric emergency procedures. In Fleisher GR, Ludwig S (eds). *Textbook of Pediatric Emergency Medicine* (3rd ed). Baltimore, Williams and Wilkins, 1993, pp 1576-1577.

Chameides L. *Textbook of Pediatric Advanced Life Support.* Dallas, American Heart Association, 1988, pp 39-41.

CHAPTER 18

James R. Harley

SUBCLAVIAN VENOUS CANNULATION

INDICATIONS

1. Central intravenous access
2. Central venous pressure (CVP) measurement
3. Swan-Ganz catheter insertion

CONTRAINDICATIONS

1. Chest compressions in progress
2. Patients less than 6 yr of age may not be able to be restrained safely for this procedure without deep sedation.

EQUIPMENT

1. Towel roll
2. Tape
3. Central line kit (introducer needle, 1% lidocaine, 22- and 27-gauge needles, 5- and 10-cc syringes, guidewire, dilator, catheter, scalpel, suture, Betadine solution, sterile towels, and heparin flush 100 U/cc of normal saline)

PROCEDURE

1. Place the patient in a supine position with a towel roll under the shoulder. Tilt the bed to a Trendelenburg position of 20 to 30 degrees. Have an assistant turn the head away from the side to be cannulated, provided the cervical spine has been cleared of possible injury (see Fig. 16–1). Wear sterile gloves and a mask.
2. Place the patient on a cardiac monitor.
3. See Chapter 14 for description of Seldinger's technique.
4. Estimate the length of the catheter to be inserted by holding it over the site of insertion, curving under the clavicle; the tip should lie over the angle of the manubrium-sternum junction.
5. Using an introducer needle attached to a syringe, enter the skin just underneath the clavicle at the junction of the middle and medial third of the clavicle. Place index finger of other hand in sternal notch. Direct the needle toward your

fingertip. The needle and syringe should be kept parallel to the frontal plane (Fig. 18-1).

6. Once blood is obtained, rotate the needle caudally so the bevel is facing down to facilitate the downward turn of the guidewire.

7. Remove the syringe. Cover the tip of the needle with a finger to prevent air entry.

8. Insert the guidewire through the needle (during exhalation if patient is not receiving positive pressure ventilation). The guidewire should advance easily without excessive force (see Fig. 14-3).

9. Advance the guidewire the estimated distance to the junction of the superior vena cava and right atrium. If a premature beat is seen or heard, withdraw the guidewire 1 cm. Monitor the patient carefully while advancing the guidewire. If the guidewire advances 2 to 4 cm past the end of the introducer needle but then fails to advance any farther, try moving the patient's head to the midline position or toward the side of insertion; then try to advance the guidewire again.

10. Obtain an x-ray film to confirm placement. If the guidewire fails to advance easily, remove it and relocate the vein with the introducer needle, and reinsert the guidewire. If the guidewire meets resistance on removal, do not apply excessive force to the guidewire; rather, remove it and the needle in tandem.

11. Advance the guidewire the estimated distance to the junction of the superior vena cava and right atrium. If a premature beat is seen or heard, withdraw the guidewire 1 cm. Monitor the patient carefully while advancing the guidewire. If the guidewire advances 2 to 4 cm past the end of the introducer needle but then fails to advance any farther, try moving the patient's head to the midline position or toward the side of insertion; then try to advance the guidewire again.

12. Remove the introducer needle. Stabilize the guidewire. Never let go of the guidewire until it is removed from the patient.

13. Make a small nick in the skin over the guidewire top to facilitate catheter entry.

14. Insert the dilator over the guidewire. Rotate the dilator with advancement to ease entry. Then remove the dilator. Be careful to avoid inadvertent advancement of the guidewire while inserting the dilator.

15. Insert the catheter over the guidewire. Take care never to let go of the guidewire (see Fig. 14-5).

16. Remove the guidewire.

17. Aspirate blood to confirm placement.

18. Connect port to IV tubing. Flush unconnected ports with heparin solution.

19. Secure catheter to skin with sutures.

20. Obtain an x-ray examination to confirm placement.

COMPLICATIONS

1. Pneumothorax
2. Pneumomediastinum
3. Hemothorax
4. Hydrothorax
5. Local site infection
6. Bacteremia/sepsis
7. Chylothorax
8. Dysrhythmia

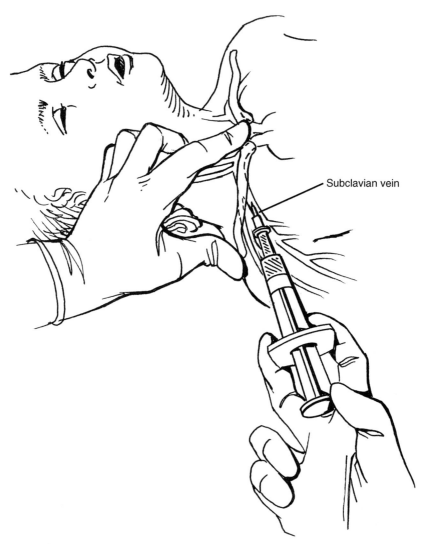

Subclavian vein

Figure 18–1. To place a subclavian catheter, enter the skin with the introducer needle attached to a syringe, at the lower margin of the clavicle at the junction of the middle third and medial third of the clavicle. Place the index finger on the sternal notch and direct the needle tip toward your finger.

9. Air embolism
10. Catheter embolism
11. Hematoma
12. Thrombosis

References

Carlson DW, Digiulio GA, Gewitz MH, et al. Illustrated techniques of pediatric emergency procedures. In Fleisher GR, Ludwig S (eds). *Textbook of Pediatric Emergency Medicine* (3rd ed). Baltimore, Williams and Wilkins, 1993, pp 1578-1579.
Chameides L. *Textbook of Pediatric Advanced Life Support.* Dallas, American Heart Association, 1988, pp 39-41.
Dronen SC. Central venous catheterization: Subclavian vein approach. In Roberts JR, Hedges JR (eds). *Clinical Procedures in Emergency Medicine* (2nd ed). Philadelphia, WB Saunders, 1991, pp 325-340.

CHAPTER 19

Steven Krug

VENOUS CUTDOWN

INDICATIONS

1. Venous cannulation when percutaneous methods fail

(**NOTE:** For those children with circulatory collapse or cardiopulmonary failure, intraosseus remains the alternative method of choice when percutaneous techniques fail.)

CONTRAINDICATIONS

1. Suspected venous injury proximal to selected site
2. Coagulopathy (relative)
3. Percutaneous access possible

EQUIPMENT

1. Betadine
2. Sterile sponges
3. Sterile field
4. Mask, gown, sterile gloves
5. Local anesthetic: 2-ml syringe, 22- and 25-gauge needles, 1% lidocaine
6. Scalpel: #11 blade
7. Soft tissue retractors (2 small rakes and/or 1 small self-retaining retractor)
8. Clamps (curved and straight mosquito)
9. Needle holder
10. Forceps (fine-toothed and smooth)
11. Scissors (suture, Metzenbaum, curved iris)
12. 3-0 silk ligatures
13. Skin suture (4-0 or 5-0 nylon or Prolene)
14. Silastic venous cutdown catheter (various gauges should be available)
15. Injectable saline, loaded into 20-cc syringe with a T connector
16. Dressing materials

PROCEDURE

1. Identify insertion site.
   a. Saphenous vein at the ankle: 1.5 cm anterior and cephalad to the medial malleolus
   (**NOTE:** This is the preferred peripheral venous cutdown site in children.)
   (See Fig. 12-3)

   b. Saphenous vein at the groin: 3 to 4 cm distal to the inguinal ligament, approximately 1 to 2 cm medial to the femoral artery
   (**NOTE:** This is the preferred central venous cutdown access site in children.)
   (See Fig. 12-3)

   c. Basilic vein at the antecubital fossa: 2 cm proximal and 2 to 3 cm lateral to the medial epicondyle
   (**NOTE:** This is the preferred venous cutdown site in the upper extremity.)
   (See Fig. 12-1)

   d. Cephalic vein at the antecubital fossa: midline at the distal flexor crease (see Fig. 12-1)
   e. Cephalic vein at the deltopectoral groove (see Fig. 12-1)
   f. External jugular vein at the posterior lateral aspect of the sternocleidomastoid muscle
   (**NOTE:** Not recommended as a cutdown access site in children)

2. Don mask, gown, and gloves.
3. Prepare insertion site with Betadine and drape with sterile field.
4. Infiltrate insertion site with 1% lidocaine.
5. Make a tranverse incision over the vein through the skin and subcutaneous tissue (Fig. 19-1*A*).
6. Isolate the vein via blunt dissection.
7. Pass two 3-0 silk ligatures beneath the vein, one each at the proximal and distal aspects of the exposed vein. Tie the distal ligature (Fig. 19-1*B*).
8. Select cannula of appropriate gauge and length.
9. Perform venotomy with #11 scalpel blade, angling the incision distally and superficially.

or

10. Cannulate vein using needle over which or through which a plastic cannula may be threaded into the vein (Fig. 19-1*C*).
11. Insert cannula into the vein, gently advancing cannula while relaxing the proximal ligature.
12. Aspirate the cannula using the 20-cc syringe and T connector filled with injectable saline. If a free flow of blood is confirmed, then flush the catheter with saline.
13. Secure cannula in the vein by tying the proximal ligature.
    (**NOTE:** Remember to reflush the cannula after tying the ligature and before closing the wound to ensure patency.)

14. Close and dress the wound.

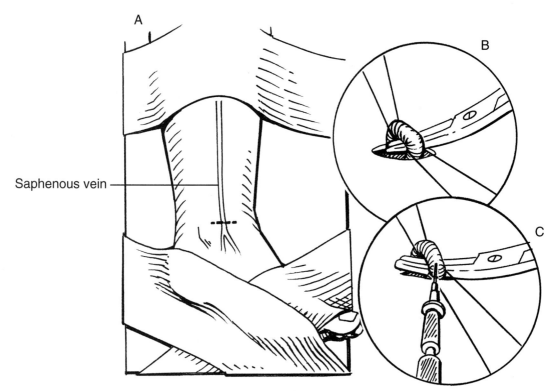

Saphenous vein

Figure 19–1. Identify the venous site and make a small transverse incision through the skin and subcutaneous tissue (*A*). Silk ligatures are used to pull the vessel into the field (inset *B*). The cannula may be introduced directly into the exposed vein (Inset *C*).

COMPLICATIONS

1. Blood loss due to injury to vascular structures
2. Local hematoma
3. Local wound infection
4. Sepsis
5. Thrombophlebitis
6. Embolization
7. Inadvertent arterial cannulation
8. Injury to adjacent structures related to site of insertion
    a. Saphenous vein at the ankle: injury to the saphenous nerve
    b. Saphenous vein at the groin: injury to lateral femoral cutaneous vein, injury to the femoral artery and nerve
    c. Basilic vein: injury to the underlying brachial artery or median nerve
    d. Cephalic vein at the antecubital fossa: injury to the lateral cutaneous nerve of the forearm
    e. External jugular vein: injury to the greater auricular nerve

References

Committee on Trauma: *Advanced Trauma Life Support Course for Physicians*. Chicago, American College of Surgeons, 1989, pp 81-83.

Dronen SC: Venous cutdown. In Roberts JR, Hedges JR (eds): *Clinical Procedures in Emergency Medicine* (2nd ed). Philadelphia, WB Saunders, 1991, pp 315-324.

Ruddy RM (ed): Illustrated techniques of pediatric emergency medicine. In Fleisher GR, Ludwig S (eds): *Textbook of Pediatric Emergency Medicine* (3rd ed). Baltimore, Williams & Wilkins, 1993, pp 1572-1573.

Vander Salm TJ: Venous cutdown. In Vander Salm TJ (ed): *Atlas of Bedside Procedures*. Boston, Little, Brown, 1979, pp 11-23.

CHAPTER 20

Jim R. Harley

ARTERIAL CUTDOWN

INDICATIONS

Need for frequent arterial blood gas assessment or continuous blood pressure monitoring when percutaneous methods have failed

CONTRAINDICATIONS

1. Impaired circulation distal to the site of insertion
2. Occlusion of the artery to be catheterized may impair circulation (i.e., abnormal Allen test)
3. Bleeding diathesis
4. Infection over site of insertion

EQUIPMENT

1. #11 or #15 scalpel blade
2. Betadine solution
3. Sterile towels
4. Silk suture ties (0-0 or 1-0)
5. Nylon suture (3-0 or 4-0)
6. Syringe (3 or 5 cc)
7. IV pressure tubing
8. 3-way stopcock
9. Mosquito hemostats
10. 20- to 24-gauge over-the-needle angiocath or 20- to 22-gauge arterial catheter
11. Needle driver for suture

PROCEDURE

Radial Artery

1. Assess collateral circulation with the Allen test (see Fig. 13-1). Occlude both the radial and ulnar arteries. The patient then squeezes his or her own hand until the hand is pale. If the patient is unable to cooperate, the hand can be squeezed by the examiner. The pressure on the ulnar artery is released. The

hand should fill with blood quickly (less than 5 sec). If it does not fill quickly, the artery should not be used.

2. The radial artery pulse is palpated proximal to the crease in the palmar surface of the wrist.
3. The site is prepped with Betadine and sterilely draped.
4. 1% lidocaine is infiltrated in the area of insertion.
5. A 2-cm horizontal incision is made through the skin just distal to the palmar transverse crease over the radial artery (Fig. 20–1A).
6. The tissue around the artery is dissected bluntly with mosquito hemostats. The direction of dissection should always be parallel to the artery.
7. The artery should be exposed for a distance of 1 cm.
8. Two silk sutures should be placed underneath the artery to aid in cannulation. (Fig. 20–1B)
9. Using an arterial or venous (over-the-needle) catheter, insert the catheter into the artery (Fig. 20–1C).
10. Attach pressure tubing to the catheter along with a 3-way stopcock.
11. The silk sutures are then removed.
12. The incision should be then closed with sutures.
13. The catheter should be sutured into place.

Posterior Tibial Artery

1. The posterior tibial artery is palpated or located by Doppler examination. It should be just posterior to the medial malleolus (Fig. 20–2).
2. Prepare the cut-down site with Betadine and infiltrate with 1% lidocaine.

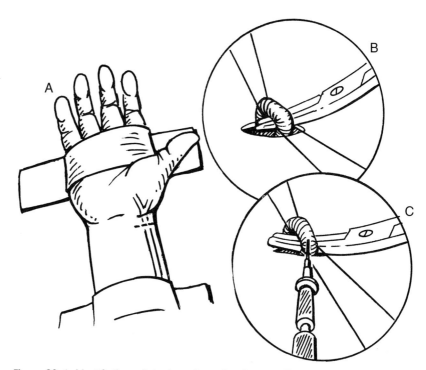

Figure 20–1. Identify the radial artery site and make a small transverse incision through the skin and subcutaneous tissue (A). Silk ligatures are used to pull the vessel into the field (inset B). The cannula may be introduced directly into the exposed vein (Inset C).

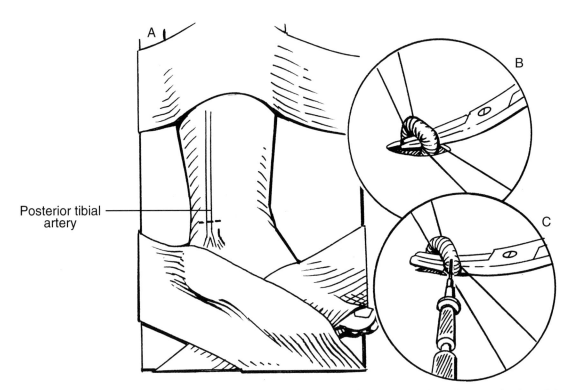

Posterior tibial
artery

Figure 20–2. Cutdown on the posterior tibial artery is performed using the technique identical to that for the radial artery. The pulse is palpated just posterior to the medial malleolus.

3. Make a 5- to 7-mm transverse incision through the skin over the artery.
4. The soft tissue over and around the artery is dissected bluntly with curved hemostats. The direction of dissection should be parallel to the artery.
5. The artery is then isolated just anterior to the vein.
6. Curved hemostats are placed underneath the vessel to isolate it.
7. A silk tie is then placed around the vessel for stabilization during cannulation.
8. The vessel is then cannulated with an angiocath or arterial catheter.
9. Remove the silk ties.
10. Once the vessel is successfully cannulated, close the incision with suture.
11. Suture the catheter to the skin.

COMPLICATIONS

1. Bleeding
2. Hematoma
3. Embolization or thrombosis of the artery
4. Local infection
5. Sepsis/bacteremia
6. Ischemia and/or infarction distal to the cannulated artery

References

Barker WJ. Arterial puncture and cannulation. In Roberts JR, Hedges JR (eds). *Clinical Procedures in Emergency Medicine* (2nd ed). Philadelphia, WB Saunders, 1991, pp 284-287.

Carlson DW, Digiulio GA, Gewitz MH, et al. Illustrated techniques of pediatric emergency procedures. In Fleisher GR, Ludwig S (eds). *Textbook of Pediatric Emergency Medicine* (3rd ed). Baltimore, Williams & Wilkins, 1993, p 1587.

CHAPTER 21

Michele Walsh-Sukys

PERCUTANEOUS INTERMEDIATE AND CENTRAL VENOUS CATHETERS

INDICATIONS

1. Prolonged venous access
2. Central venous placement needed to deliver high-concentration dextrose parenteral nutrition

CONTRAINDICATIONS

1. Bacteremia
2. Absence of suitable sites

EQUIPMENT

1. Silastic percutaneous catheter in lengths of 5 to 8 cm for intermediate placements, or 20 to 30 cm for central placement (Fig. 21–1)
2. T connector
3. Two 1-ml syringes
4. Heparinized flush solutions
5. Betadine prep solution
6. Alcohol
7. Tourniquet or rubber band
8. Sterile towels
9. Steri-Strips
10. Transparent dressing
11. Tape
12. Sterile gloves
13. Masks
14. Caps

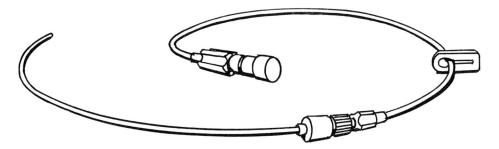

Figure 21–1. Various manufacturers provide small Silastic catheters to be used for long-term venous access.

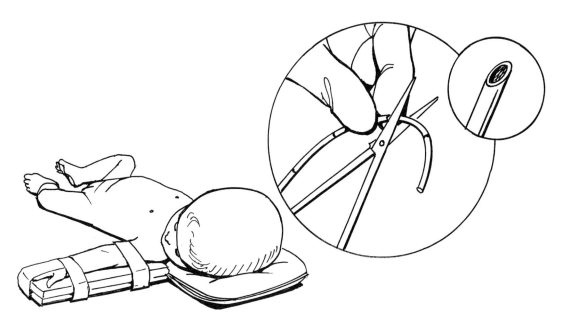

Figure 21–2. Position the patient supine with a roll between the scapulae. Prepare the catheter according to the manufacturer's directions. Some catheters may have to be cut to the correct length.

TECHNIQUE

1. Optimal placement requires the assistance of two individuals.
2. Don caps and masks. Wash hands.
3. Select a suitable vein. Any vein may be used, but the greatest success is achieved with the basilic, cephalic, axillary, or saphenous veins.
4. Measure the distance from the selected site to the approximate level of the right atrium. Position the patient supine with roll between scapulae to lift clavicular areas. Cut the catheter to the desired length, ensuring a level on the end (Fig. 21-2).
5. Triple prep selected site with Betadine, allowing solution to remain on the skin for a minimum of 30 sec. Wipe off Betadine with alcohol or sterile water.
6. Assistant applies tourniquet or rubberband above desired insertion site.
7. Don sterile gloves. Prepare sterile field around site with sterile towels.

Standard Introducer Technique

8. A 19-gauge butterfly needle from which the tubing has been removed may be used as an introducer. Various commercial manufacturers also provide kits containing both the introducer needle and the catheter.
9. Insert the needle into the selected vein until free-flowing blood return is obtained.
10. Using smooth forceps, grasp the Silastic catheter very close to the tip, and feed the catheter through the introducer needle to the desired length (Fig. 21-3).
11. Place gloved finger over the catheter site above the needle. Keeping the needle parallel with the skin to avoid severing the catheter, slowly withdraw the introducer needle (Figs. 21-4 and 21-5).

Split Needle Introducer Technique

12. Follow steps 1–7 above.
13. Prime catheter with saline. Remove needle protector. Grasp the wing assembly firmly.
14. Insert the introducer needle assembly into the vein. Confirm entry by observing the flashback of blood around the needle or into the catheter. This may take 2 to 3 sec (Fig. 21-6).
15. Release the tourniquet.
16. Stabilize the introducer needle to maintain position in the vein. Feed the catheter through the needle using either your fingers or smooth forceps.
17. Slowly back the needle out of the vein leaving the catheter in position.
18. If in place, remove the clip from the wings. Using both hands grasp opposite sides of the wings and spread the two halves until the needle peels apart. It is important to keep the needle parallel to the skin to avoid severing the catheter (Fig. 21-7).
19. Some catheters are enclosed in a sterile sleeve. Remove the sleeve carefully after the tip is advanced to the desired level.
20. If present, remove stylet, connect primed T connector, and flush the catheter.

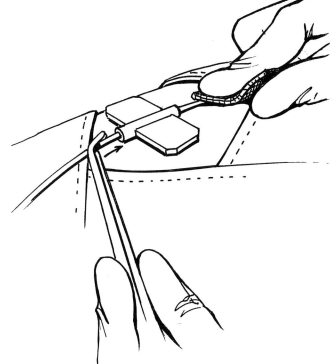

Figure 21–3. Insert the introducer needle into the vein at a very flat angle. Using smooth forceps, advance the catheter through the needle.

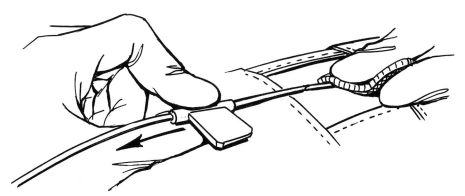

Figure 21–4. Hold the needle parallel with the skin to avoid severing the catheter, and slowly withdraw the needle over the catheter. When the needle clears the skin, secure the catheter by trapping it with your finger at the skin exit site.

Stabilizing and Caring for the Catheter

1. Secure catheter in place with Steri-Strips.
2. Confirm catheter tip placement. This may be aided by the injection of 0.3 ml of a contrast agent.
3. Apply sterile transparent dressing over the insertion site. The dressing is usually inspected daily but is changed only when it becomes nonocclusive (Fig. 21-8).
4. Infuse intravenous (IV) fluids containing heparin (1 U/ml) to promote catheter patency.
5. Policies regarding infusion of blood products via the percutaneous central catheter vary widely between institutions. Many units discourage the administration of blood via this route, but evidence supporting this practice is lacking.

Salvaging a Clotted Catheter

1. Urokinase, a thrombolytic agent, may be used to restore the patency of a percutaneous central catheter.
2. As soon as a clot is detected, administer urokinase (5000 IU/ml) 0.1 ml into the line.
3. Allow the urokinase to remain in place for 5 min and then attempt to gently aspirate both the urokinase and the clot. Repeat attempts every 5 min for 30 min.
4. If patency is not restored after 30 min, repeat step 3. If the second attempt is not successful after an additional 30 min, the catheter must be removed.
5. When patency is restored, aspirate and discard 0.2 ml of blood to ensure complete removal of drug and clot.
6. Flush the line with normal saline and reconnect IV tubing.

COMPLICATIONS

1. During line placement
   a. Intra-arterial insertion: Remove the line and hold pressure for 3 to 5 min.
   b. Inability to thread the catheter past the introducer needle
      (1) Generally, if this occurs, the introducer needle tip has passed through the lumen and into the posterior wall. Remove the introducer needle and try again at another site.
      (2) Occasionally the introducer needle may be correctly placed into the lumen, yet the catheter's progress is impeded by contacting the vessel wall. Reorienting the introducer needle (slightly to the right or left) may overcome this.
   c. Severing the catheter during withdrawal of the introducer needle: If this occurs, immediately apply pressure on the vessel above the insertion site in an attempt to limit the proximal migration of the catheter. Grasp any portion of the catheter remaining outside the body and slowly withdraw. If no portion of the catheter is visible, an open venotomy must be performed to extract the catheter.
2. Others
   a. Infection
   b. Infiltration
   c. Mechanical complications

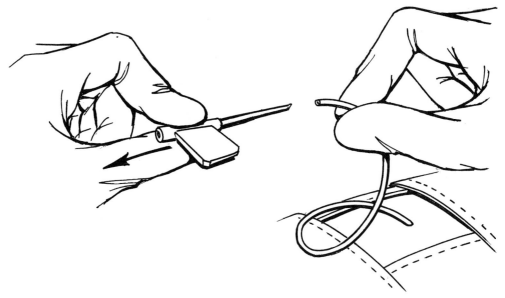

Figure 21–5. Slowly remove the needle the remainder of the distance over the catheter.

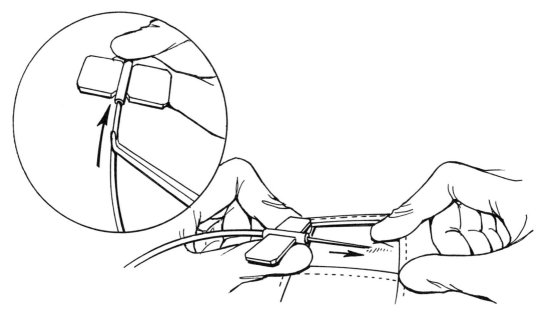

Figure 21–6. Insert the introducer needle assembly into the vein until a flashback of blood is observed. Feed the catheter through the introducer needle using your fingers or smooth forceps.

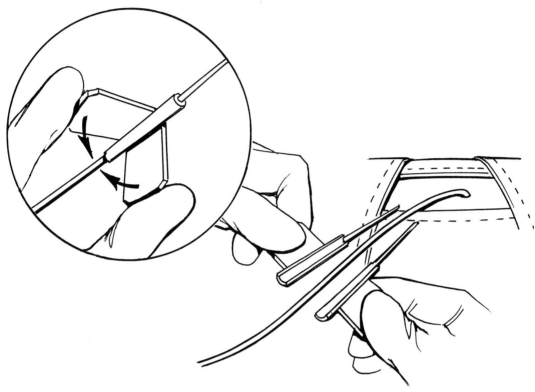

Figure 21–7. After slowly backing the needle out of the vein, follow the manufacturer's directions to split the two wings of the introducer needle, and then use two hands to gently peel the two wings apart.

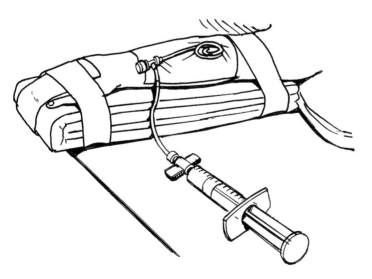

Figure 21–8. Apply a sterile transparent dressing over the catheter.

(1) Catheter occlusion by calcium phosphate crystals. These usually have been seen in patients receiving fluids containing concentrations of calcium exceeding 20 mEq/l. A white precipitate may be seen in the line. Urokinase is not efficacious in this setting.

(2) Accidental catheter dislodgement

(3) Ruptured catheters: Attempts to flush the catheter too rapidly or too aggressively may result in rupture. A technique to repair catheters that rupture this way has been described. However, because of concerns about possible bacterial contamination of catheters that are intended to have long dwell times, ruptured catheters are usually removed rather than repaired.

References

Dolcourt JL, Bose CL. Percutaneous insertion of Silastic central venous catheters in newborn infants. Pediatrics 70:484, 1982.

Durand M, Ramanathan R, Martinelli B, Tolentino M. Prospective evaluation of percutaneous central venous silastic catheters in newborn infants with birthweights of 510-3920 grams. Pediatrics 78:245, 1986.

Reynolds, J. Comparison of percutaneous venous catheters and Teflon catheters for intravenous therapy in neonates. Neonatal Network 12:84-90, 1993.

CHAPTER 22

Steven Krug

PULMONARY ARTERY CATHETERIZATION

INDICATIONS

1. Need for precise hemodynamic data collection and monitoring in the critically ill child, including pulmonary artery pressure, cardiac output, oxygen delivery, right ventricular end-systolic and end-diastolic volumes and ejection fractions, mixed-venous oxygen saturation

CONTRAINDICATIONS

1. Coagulopathy (relative)

EQUIPMENT

1. Betadine
2. Sterile sponges
3. Sterile field
4. Mask, gown, sterile gloves
5. Local anesthetic: 1% lidocaine
6. Scalpel: #11 blade
7. Sheath introducer tray, including angiocatheter or other over-the-needle catheter, appropriate-sized J wire, vessel introducer (vessel dilator and catheter sheath)
8. Pulmonary artery catheter

   7 Fr > 18 kg
   5 Fr < 18 kg

9. Heparinized saline (1000 u/100 ml)
10. Syringes (10 cc, 1 cc)
11. Needle holder
12. Forceps (fine-toothed and smooth)
13. Scissors (suture, Metzenbaum, curved iris)
14. Suture (3-0 or 4-0 silk)
15. Dressing materials
16. Sterile saline and small sterile specimen cup
17. Monitor/defibrillator

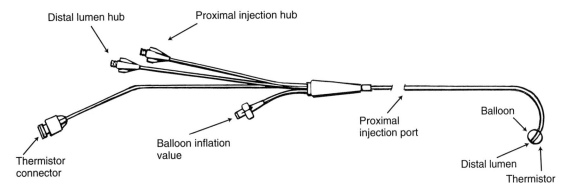

Figure 22–1. Flush all ports of the pulmonary artery catheter and test the balloon for patency.

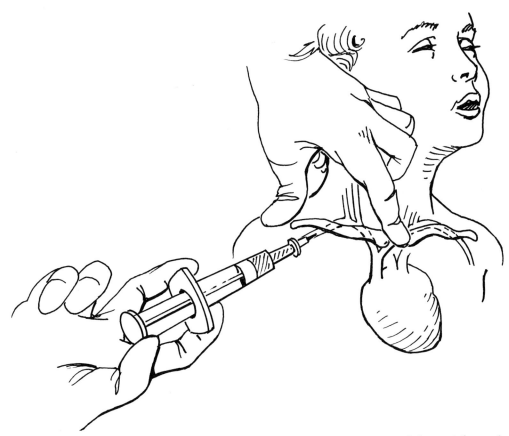

Figure 22–2. Insert the catheter into the desired vein. The subclavian vein is one of the most frequently used sites.

PROCEDURE

1. Connect the patient to a dynamic cardiorespiratory monitor and place in a position that supports catheter insertion (10 to 20 degrees Trendelenburg). (See Fig. 16-1)
2. Identify insertion site: right or left femoral vein, right internal jugular vein, left internal jugular vein, left subclavian vein, right subclavian vein, right or left external jugular vein, right or left basilic vein.
3. Don mask, gown, and gloves.
4. Examine catheter tray. Make sure that the component parts are of compatible size. Flush all ports of the pulmonary artery catheter with heparinized saline (Fig. 22-1). Test catheter balloon by injecting air with balloon submerged in sterile saline.
5. Prepare insertion site with Betadine and drape with sterile field.
6. Infiltrate insertion site with 1% lidocaine.
7. Attach 10-cc syringe to the angiocatheter. Insert catheter into the desired vein. Confirm catheter placement via free flow of blood into the syringe.
8. Advance the catheter slightly farther into the vein and remove the needle and syringe apparatus, leaving the catheter in place (Fig. 22-2).
9. Insert the J wire into the angiocatheter. This should advance easily. Monitor the patient for ECG changes (if suspected, withdraw the wire 2 cm) (Fig. 22-3). Insertion should also allow for a sufficient length of wire at the surface greater then the length of the pulmonary artery catheter.
10. If the wire fails to advance easily, remove the wire and reconfirm the placement of the angiocatheter.
11. With the J wire in place, remove the catheter, keeping the position of the wire unchanged (Fig. 22-4A).
12. Make a small incision in the skin adjacent to the wire with the scalpel blade. Avoid cutting the wire (Fig. 22-4B).
13. Advance the introducer (both the dilator and vessel sheath) over the wire, into the vein. Take care not to allow the inadvertent advancement of the wire into the patient. This can be ensured by maintaining control of the wire separate from the insertion of the introducer (Fig. 22-5).
14. Remove the J wire.
15. Remove the dilator leaving the sheath in place.
16. Insert the pulmonary artery catheter into the introducer sleeve, advance to a central venous position.
17. Attach pressure monitoring devices to the catheter. The position of the catheter can be determined by pressure waveforms.
18. Catheter may be advanced through the right heart and into the pulmonary artery. This may be accomplished with or without inflation of the balloon.
19. Confirm placement of the catheter using pressure waveform data (Fig. 22-6). With balloon inflated, one should have a pulmonary artery wedge pressure form (lower pressure and flattened wave amplitudes compared to pulmonary artery tracings). Balloon deflation should cause a prompt return to pulmonary artery tracing. Further confirmation may be obtained with a chest x-ray examination.
20. Secure catheter with suture.
21. Apply dressing.
22. Obtain portable chest x-ray examination to confirm placement and to rule out hemothorax or pneumothorax.

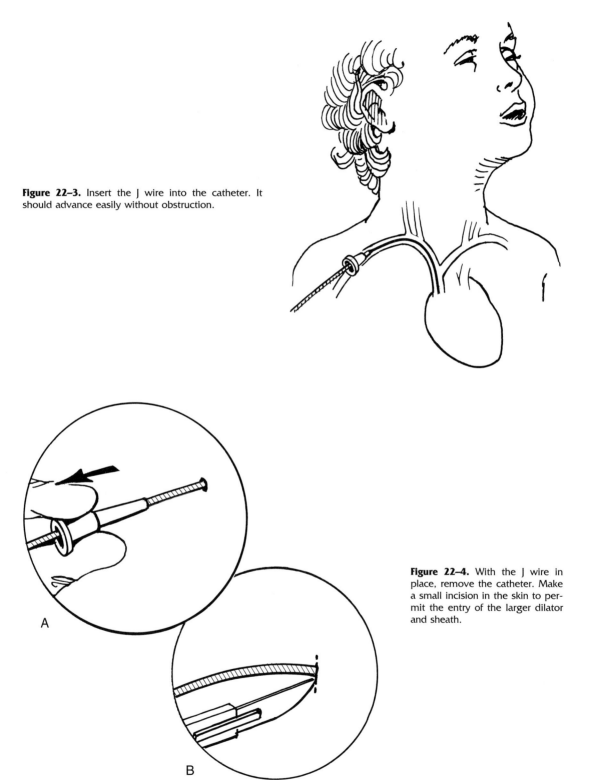

Figure 22–3. Insert the J wire into the catheter. It should advance easily without obstruction.

A

B

Figure 22–4. With the J wire in place, remove the catheter. Make a small incision in the skin to permit the entry of the larger dilator and sheath.

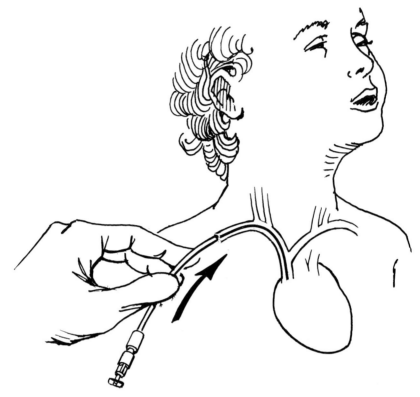

Figure 22–5. Advance the introducer over the wire, being very careful not to permit the wire to move.

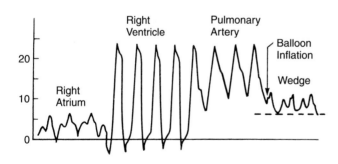

Figure 22–6. Confirm placement of the catheter by observing pressure waveforms.

COMPLICATIONS

1. Blood loss due to injury to vascular structures
2. Local hematoma
3. Local wound infection
4. Sepsis
5. Thrombophlebitis
6. Thromboembolization
7. Inadvertent arterial cannulation
8. Arrhythmia
9. Pneumothorax (subclavian or internal jugular approach)
10. Hemothorax
11. Cardiac valvular damage or traumatic endocarditis
12. Rupture or perforation of pulmonary artery
13. Cardiac tamponade
14. Pulmonary artery infarction or hemorrhage
15. Air embolism
16. Knotting or kinking of the catheter
17. Misinterpretation of data collected

References

Fitzpatrick GF: Pulmonary artery catheterization. In Vander Salm TJ (ed): *Atlas of Bedside Procedures.* Boston, Little, Brown, 1979; pp 105-117.
Katz RW, Pollack MM, Weibly RE: Pulmonary artery catheterization in pediatric intensive care. Adv Pediatr 30:169-191, 1984.
Martin GR, Holley DG: Cardiovascular monitoring and evaluation. In Holbrook PR (ed): Textbook of Pediatric Critical Care. Philadelphia, WB Saunders, 1993, pp 259-278.
Pope J: Pulmonary artery catheters. In Blumer JB (ed): *A Practical Guide to Pediatric Intensive Care* (3rd ed). St Louis, Mosby-Year Book, 1990, pp 830-837.
Swan HJC, Ganz W: Use of balloon flotation catheters in critically ill patients. Surg Clin North Am 55:501-520, 1975.
Tabata BK, Kirsch JR, Rogers MC: Diagnostic tests and technology for pediatric intensive care. In Rogers MC (ed): *Textbook of Pediatric Intensive Care.* Baltimore, Williams & Wilkins, 1987, pp 1410-1415.

CHAPTER 23

Michele Walsh-Sukys

UMBILICAL VENOUS CATHETERIZATION

INDICATIONS

1. Emergency vascular access for resuscitation in a neonate
2. Access for exchange transfusion in a neonate
3. Central venous pressure monitoring in a neonate

CONTRAINDICATION

1. Anomalies of the umbilicus and abdominal wall are relative contraindications

EQUIPMENT

1. Sterile drapes
2. Sterile gown, cap, mask, and gloves
3. Tape measure
4. Betadine solution
5. Umbilical tie tape
6. Scalpel
7. Two Kelly clamps
8. Two iris forceps with teeth
9. Two straight forceps
10. Flush solution
11. 3-way stopcock
12. Two 3-ml syringes
13. Polyvinyl chloride or Silastic catheters in various appropriate sizes (preterm, 5 Fr; term, 8 Fr)
14. Needle driver
15. Absorbable suture
16. Strong light source
17. Graph to determine appropriate depth of insertion (Fig. 23-1)

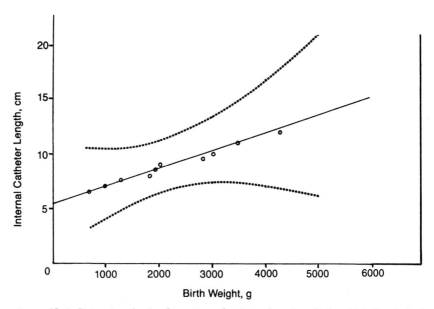

Figure 23–1. Determine depth of insertion of catheter based on birthweight. The desired position is just above the diaphragm with the tip in the inferior vena cava or at the junction with the right atrium. (Modified from Shukla H and Ferrara A. Rapid estimation of insertional length of umbilical catheters in newborns. Am J Dis Child 140:786–788, 1986. Copyright 1986, American Medical Association.)

TECHNIQUE

1. Determine the appropriate depth of line insertion using either the total body length or birthweight (Fig. 23-1). In an emergency, the line is inserted until blood return is obtained. Another rule of thumb is to insert approximately 5 cm in a preterm baby, and 10 cm in a term baby. The desired location of the catheter tip is in the inferior vena cava (IVC) either below the portal system or at the IVC and right atrial junction.

2. Prepare the catheter by placing a 3-way stopcock on the end of the catheter and filling the catheter with a sterile saline or heparin flush solution (1 U/ml) (Fig. 23-2A, B).

3. Tie the base of the umbilicus with umbilical tie tape, taking care to avoid the abdominal wall skin.

4. Place a cloth or disposable diaper over the neonate's thighs and restrain the baby by placing tape across the baby's legs and the bed.

5. Prepare the umbilicus and abdominal wall with Betadine using sterile technique.

6. Don sterile gown and gloves and drape the baby's trunk and legs, leaving the umbilicus exposed. Ensure that the baby's head and endotracheal tube are visible to an observer during the procedure to avoid endotracheal tube occlusion or dislodgment.

7. Sever the umbilical cord with the scalpel at a 90-degree angle about 1 cm above the abdominal wall.

8. Identify two thick-walled arteries and a single thin-walled vein (Fig. 23-3).

9. Stabilize the umbilical stump by grasping the Wharton's jelly with two Kelly clamps.

10. Gently dilate the vein with the curved iris forceps. Insert the closed forceps into the vein and then gently open them. Repeat this maneuver three or four times. Remove any blood clots found (Fig. 23-3).

11. When the lumen is opened, the assistant gently grasps the venous wall with two curved forceps on opposite sides of the vessel. This will stabilize the artery and prevent it from sliding away from the catheter during insertion.

12. Grasp the catheter approximately 0.5 cm above the tip with the straight forceps and gently insert the tip into the vessel lumen (Fig. 23-4).

13. Move the forceps back up the catheter in 1-cm increments and gently advance the catheter forward.

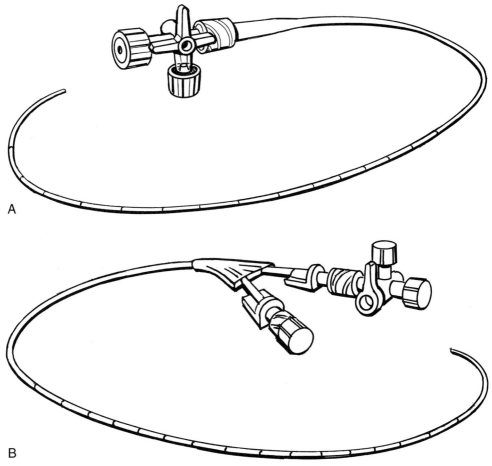

A

B

Figure 23–2. Prepare catheter by placing a 3-way stopcock and flushing with saline. Catheters are available as both single and double lumens.

Figure 23–3. Identify the thin-walled umbilical vein and dilate it gently with smooth forceps. Visualize and remove any clots present.

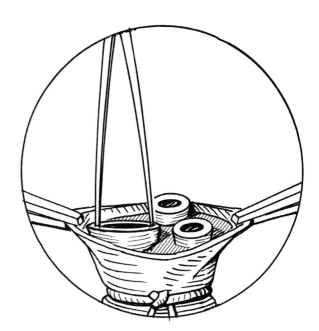

14. Suture the catheter in place securely to the umbilical stump. One technique to prevent catheter movement is to use a self-retaining suture; that is, one that becomes tighter whenever any traction is placed on the catheter. Begin the self-retaining stitch by securing the suture to the umbilical stump near the exit site of the catheter. Some operators like to place a purse string suture around the umbilicus to function as a secondary means to achieve hemostasis whereas others prefer to begin with a single through-and-through stitch. Secure the stitch with a square knot and remove the needle, leaving long segments of suture on either side of the knot (tails). Grasp one tail and encircle the tip of the needle driver two times, moving toward the catheter (Fig. 23-5A). Place the needle driver and the free end of the same tail on opposite sides of the catheter and pull the free end through the loops (inset *B*). Repeat this same movement on the opposite side using the other tail. Repeat both steps again; this will yield four loops on the catheter (inset *C-E*). Complete the stitch by tying a square knot with the two suture ends (inset *F*).

15. Ensure correct catheter position by radiograph. On an anteroposterior radiograph a catheter placed in the umbilical artery will descend before turning cephalad, whereas a venous catheter will go immediately cephalad. These two can be further distinguished on a lateral radiograph: the aorta lies just anterior to the vertebrae, whereas the vein tracks in the anterior abdominal wall.

16. One may wish to secure the catheter further by forming a bridge with tape. In very low birthweight neonates, the skin can be protected from the tape with Stomahesive material and the tape applied to this (Fig. 23-6).

17. A final useful marker is to place a piece of tape across the catheter immediately above the umbilicus. This ensures that catheter movement can be detected readily.

18. A catheter should *never* be advanced once the sterile drape is removed.

COMPLICATIONS

1. Complications resulting from malposition of an intraluminal catheter
   a. Heart: Cardiac arrythmias may be produced by catheters malpositioned in the heart. In addition, catheters that extend into the right atrium may erode, producing pericardial effusion and/or cardiac tamponade.
   b. Great vessels: Umbilical venous catheter may be advanced too vigorously and may pass out of the right atrium and into the superior vena cava or across the foramen ovale and into the left atrium.
   c. Portal system: Thrombosis of the hepatic veins has been associated with infusion of hypertonic solutions into the portal system. This may lead to hepatic infarction and/or later portal hypertension.
2. Thromboembolic events
3. Infection

Figure 23–4. Insert the catheter gently into the vein lumen.

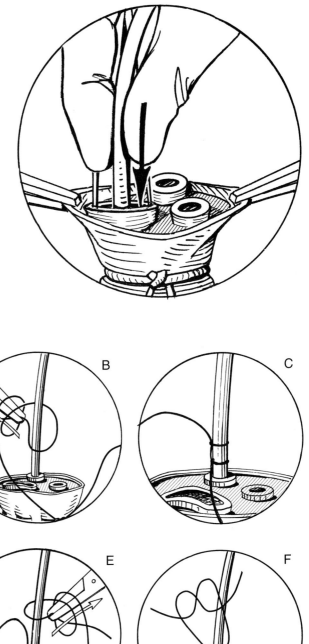

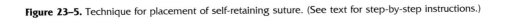

Figure 23–5. Technique for placement of self-retaining suture. (See text for step-by-step instructions.)

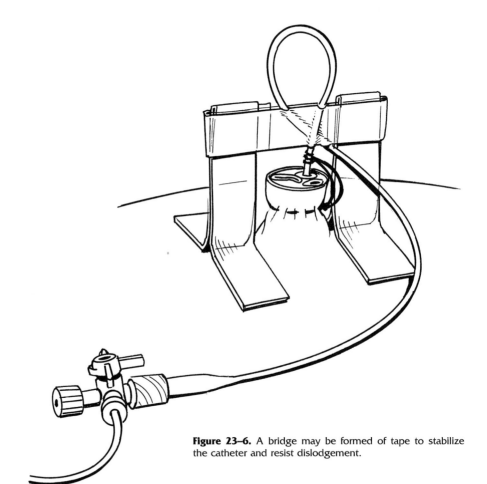

Figure 23–6. A bridge may be formed of tape to stabilize the catheter and resist dislodgement.

References

Baker DH, Berdon WE, James LS. Proper localization of umbilical catheter placement by lateral roentgenograms. Pediatrics 43:34, 1969.

Dunn P. Localization of the umbilical catheter position by post mortem measurements. Arch Dis Child 41:69, 1966.

Lauridsen UB, Enk B, Gammeltoft A. Oesophageal varices as a late complication of neonatal umbilical vein catheterization. Acta Pediatr Scand 67:633, 1978.

Savani RC, Valentini RP, Mimouni F. Pericardial effusion as a complication of umbilical venous catheterization. J Perinatol 10:443, 1990.

Shukla H, Ferrara A. Rapid estimation of insertional length of umbilical catheters in newborns. Am J Dis Child 140:786–788, 1986.

CHAPTER 24

Michele Walsh-Sukys

UMBILICAL ARTERIAL CATHETERIZATION

INDICATIONS

1. Monitoring blood pressure
2. Monitoring arterial blood gases when in supplemental oxygen
3. May be considered as an access and infusion site in all neonates with birthweight <1.0 kg in whom other access sites carry substantial risk
4. May be used as an alternative site of fluid administration when attempts at venous access are unsuccessful

CONTRAINDICATIONS

1. Anomalies of the umbilicus and abdominal wall are relative contraindications
2. Vascular impairment in the lower extremities and buttocks

EQUIPMENT

1. Sterile drapes
2. Sterile gown, cap, mask, and gloves
3. Tape measure
4. Betadine solution
5. Umbilical tie tape
6. Scalpel
7. Two Kelly clamps
8. Two iris forceps with teeth
9. Two straight forceps
10. Flush solution
11. 3-way stopcock
12. Two 3-ml syringes
13. Polyvinyl chloride or Silastic catheters in various sizes appropriate to birthweight (birthweight <750 gm, 2.5 Fr; 750–1750 gm, 3 Fr; >1750 gm, 5 Fr)
14. Needle driver
15. Absorbable suture
16. Strong light source
17. Graphs to determine appropriate depth of insertion (Figs. 24–1, 24–2, 24–3)

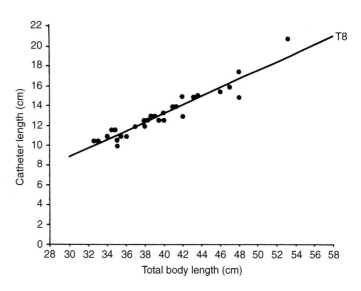

Figure 24–1. Graph depicts the appropriate depth of catheter insertion in the umbilical artery to achieve placement at thoracic vertebra 8, based on total body length. (Used with permission. Rosenfeld W, Biagtan J, Schaeffer H, et al. A new graph for insertion of umbilical artery catheters. J Pediatr 96:735–737, 1980.)

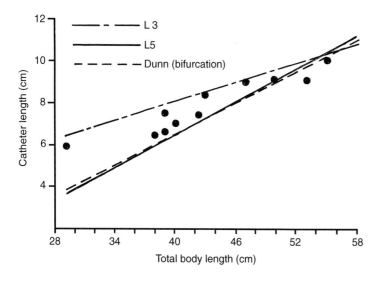

Figure 24–2. Graph depicts the appropriate depth of catheter insertion in the umbilical artery to achieve placement at lumbar vertebrae 3 to 5, based on total body length. (Used with permission. Rosenfeld W, Estrada R, Jhaveri R, et al. Evaluation of graphs for insertion of umbilical artery catheters below the diaphragm. J Pediatr 98:627–628, 1981.)

TECHNIQUE

1. Determine the appropriate depth of line insertion, using either the total body length or the birthweight (Figs. 24-1, 24-2, 24-3).
2. Prepare the catheter by placing a 3-way stopcock on the end of the catheter, and fill the catheter with a sterile saline or heparin flush solution (1 U/ml) (see Fig. 23-2).
3. Tie the base of the umbilicus with umbilical tie tape taking care to avoid the abdominal wall skin.
4. Place a cloth or disposable diaper over the neonate's thighs and restrain the baby by placing tape across the baby's legs and the bed.
5. Prepare the umbilicus and abdominal wall with Betadine, using sterile technique.
6. Don sterile gown and gloves, and drape the baby's trunk and legs leaving the umbilicus exposed. Ensure that the baby's head and endotracheal tube are visible to an observer during the procedure to avoid endotracheal tube occlusion or dislodgement.
7. Sever the umbilical cord with the scalpel at a 90-degree angle about 1 cm above the abdominal wall.
8. Identify two thick-walled arteries and a single thin-walled vein (Fig. 24-4).
9. Stabilize the umbilical stump by grasping the Wharton's jelly with two Kelly clamps.
10. Gently dilate the artery with the curved iris forceps. Insert the closed forceps into the artery and then gently open them. Repeat this manuever three or four times (Fig. 24-4).
11. When the lumen is opened, the assistant gently grasps the arterial wall with two curved forceps on opposite sides of the vessel. This will stabilize the artery and prevent it from sliding away from the catheter during insertion.
12. Grasp the catheter approximately 0.5 cm above the tip with the straight forceps and gently insert the tip into the vessel lumen (Fig. 24-5).
13. Move the forceps back up the catheter in 1-cm increments and gently advance the catheter forward.
14. If resistance is met at any point, gentle pressure may be held on the catheter at that point, but no attempt should be made to advance beyond the resistance unless the resistance resolves. Resistance may be produced by vasospasm, which may spontaneously resolve. Alternatively, it may be encountered when the catheter has been introduced to the 3- to 5-cm mark at the point where the umbilical artery enters the iliac artery and the catheter must negotiate an acute turn. Vigorous attempts to advance the catheter past resistance at this point may result in perforation. If the resistance does not spontaneously resolve, it is most prudent to abandon the attempt at placement and try again in the other artery.
15. Advance the catheter to the predetermined appropriate depth to result in either a "high" line (thoracic vertebrae 8-11) or a "low" line (lumbar vertebrae 3-5). These positions avoid the major vascular branches from the aorta.
16. Suture catheter in place securely to the umbilical stump (see Fig. 23-5). One technique to prevent catheter movement is to use a self-retaining suture; that is, one that becomes tighter whenever any traction is placed on the catheter. Begin the self-retaining stitch by securing the suture to the umbilical stump near the exit site of the catheter. Some surgeons place a purse string suture around the umbilicus to function as a secondary means to achieve hemostasis, whereas others prefer to begin with a single through-and-through stitch. Secure

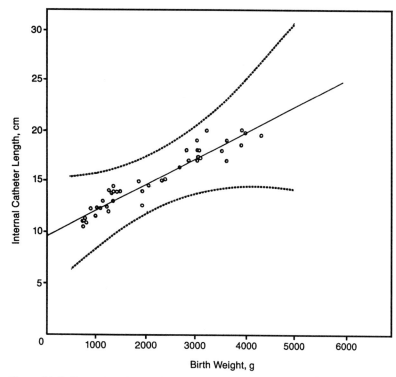

Figure 24–3. Determine depth of insertion of catheter into the umbilical artery based on birthweight. The graph predicts placement between thoracic vertebrae 6 and 10. (Modified from Shukla H and Ferrara A. Rapid estimation of insertional length of umbilical catheters in newborns. Am J Dis Child 140: 786–788, 1986. Copyright 1986, American Medical Association.)

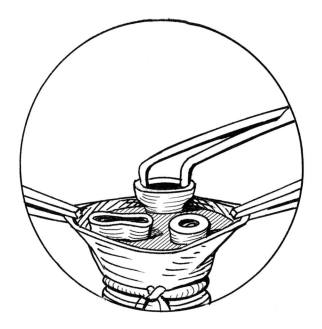

Figure 24–4. Identify two thick-walled arteries and one thin-walled vein. The artery may be dilated by inserting the closed forceps into the lumen and then spreading them open. Otherwise, grasp each side of the vessel with a forceps and open gently.

the stitch with a square knot and remove the needle leaving long segments of suture on either side of the knot (tails). Grasp one tail and encircle the tip of the needle driver two times, moving toward the catheter (inset *A*). Place the needle driver and the free end of the same tail on opposite sides of the catheter and pull the free end through the loops (inset *B*). Repeat this same movement on the opposite side using the other tail. Repeat both steps again, which will yield four loops on the catheter (insets *C-E*). Complete the stitch by tying a square knot with the two suture ends (inset *F*).

17. Ensure correct catheter position by radiograph. On an anteroposterior radiograph a catheter placed in the umbilical artery will descend before turning cephalad, whereas a venous catheter will go immediately cephalad. These two can be further distinguished on a lateral radiograph: The aorta lies just anterior to the vertebrae, whereas the vein tracks in the anterior abdominal wall.

18. One may wish to secure the catheter further by forming a bridge with tape. In very low birthweight neonates, the skin can be protected from the tape with Stomahesive material and the tape applied to this (see Fig. 23-6).

19. A final useful marker is to place a piece of tape across the catheter immediately above the umbilicus. This ensures that catheter movement can be detected readily.

20. A catheter should *never* be advanced once the sterile drape is removed.

COMPLICATIONS

1. The vast majority of complications arise from failure to exert adequate caution and time to dilate the umbilical artery at the beginning of catheter insertion. This can lead to:
   a. Vessel perforation (Figs. 24-6 and 24-7*A*)
   b. Dissection of the tunica intima (false tracking) (Fig. 24-7*B*)
   c. Avulsion of the tunica intima (false tracking) (Fig. 24-7*C*)
   All of these may be suspected during catheter placement when resistance is encountered within 1 to 3 cm of catheter placement or if a "pop" is felt. If any of these are encountered the safest course of action is to remove the catheter from the affected artery and try again in the opposite vessel.

2. Vessel perforation posterior to the bladder: The umbilical artery follows an inferior course and descends behind the bladder, and then turns nearly 180 degrees to join the iliac artery, then the femoral artery, and then the abdominal aorta (see Fig. 24-6). At the point at which the umbilical artery turns, the catheter must negotiate an acute angle. Resistance may be encountered at this point, which is at approximately 5-cm catheter depth. Vigorous attempts to advance the catheter may result in perforation of the posterior wall of the umbilical artery and retroperitoneal hematoma formation (see Fig. 24-8). Bleeding into this concealed space may be life threatening and requires surgical exploration to correct. Ultrasound may be used to confirm the diagnosis.

3. Complications resulting from malposition of an intraluminal catheter:
   a. The catheter may turn and track inferiorly down the iliac artery occluding circulation to the leg. Alternatively, the vessel may be in spasm. Immediately following catheter placement, perfusion to the toes of both legs must be assessed. If any evidence of cyanosis is visible, the catheter must be pulled back to a more central position immediately. If one extremity is dusky, vasospasm may be diagnosed and treated by warming the contralateral extremity (wrapping the other extremity with a diaper warmed with tap water

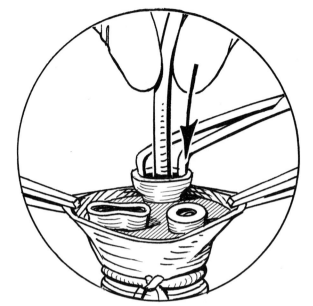

Figure 24–5. Insert the catheter gently into the arterial lumen. Force should never be used to advance the catheter or vessel perforation may result.

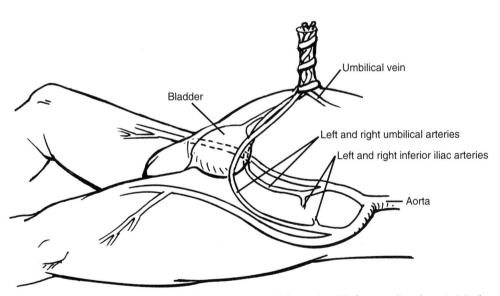

Umbilical vein

Bladder

Left and right umbilical arteries

Left and right inferior iliac arteries

Aorta

Figure 24–6. The umbilical arteries travel down the anterior abdominal wall before traveling down to join the inferior iliac arteries. Difficulty may be encountered when passing a catheter around this acute turn.

works well for this). Warming of the well-perfused extremity induces reflex vasodilation in the affected extremity. If cyanosis persists for more than 5 min, the catheter should be removed.

b. Occlusion to the gluteal artery can lead to necrosis of the buttocks: Involvement of the gluteus maximus can lead to major impairment of ambulation later in life. Radiographs will identify malposition in this vessel.

c. Occlusion of a spinal artery may occur when an otherwise well-placed catheter errantly enters any of the spinal arteries arising from the aorta. Again radiographs will identify any malposition.

d. Occlusion of the renal arteries or celiac trunk: Catheters positioned between thoracic vertebrae 11 and lumbar vertebra 2 may impinge on the flow of blood into these major vessels. Malposition may be detected radiographically.

e. Placement at the patent ductus arteriosus (PDA): A catheter placed at thoracic vertebrae 4 may be positioned at the PDA, which may contribute to ductal patency.

f. Placement of the catheter too far superiorly will lead it to advance up the aorta into the left ventricle or vessels serving the arms, neck, or head. Left ventricular placement may precipitate arrhythmias, whereas positioning in more distal vessels may lead to vascular occlusion. These can be prevented by predetermining the depth of catheter insertion and can be detected radiographically.

4. Emboli related to catheters

a. Air or debris may be introduced whenever the catheter is infused on or flushed. Meticulous attention is needed to ensure that air is not introduced. Emboli may be seen in any distal circulatory bed. The most severe consequences of emboli are seen when they involve the coronary circulation, (which may lead to myocardial infarction), the cerebral circulation (which may produce stroke), the renal circulation (with infarction and hypertension), or the gut circulation (leading to necrotizing enterocolitis).

b. High catheters are more frequently associated with embolic events producing seizures, whereas low catheters more frequently are associated with embolic events involving the lower extremity. Necrotizing enterocolitis is equally common in both groups.

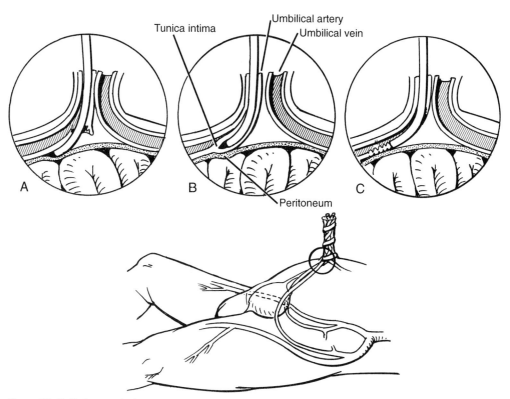

Figure 24–7. Catheter misplacement may arise through a number of different mechanisms. *A,* The posterior wall of the artery may be perforated by the catheter. This may lead to hematomas at the base of the umbilical stump or in the anterior abdominal wall. *B,* The catheter may dissect through the layers of intima creating a false track and the potential for aneurysm formation. *C,* The intima may be avulsed from the endothelium and pushed ahead of the catheter.

CHAPTER 25

Steven Krug

INTRAOSSEUS INFUSION

INDICATIONS

1. As a means for rapid, temporary vascular access for children with circulatory collapse or cardiopulmonary failure when more routine methods of vascular access (e.g., percutaneous venous access) have failed. The threshold for the procedure in this scenario has been suggested to be three failed attempts, or 90 sec elapsed.
2. As a primary means of vascular access for children suffering cardiopulmonary arrest

CONTRAINDICATIONS

1. Should not be used as a method for "routine" vascular access in nonemergent settings
2. Relative contraindications for older children and adults
3. Not for use as a means for long-term vascular access
4. Should not be performed on a fractured bone or, ideally, on a bone with a previous failed attempt

EQUIPMENT

1. Commercially available intraosseus needle (Fig. 25-1)
2. Betadine
3. 20-cc syringe
4. Intravenous (IV) tubing and fluids, stopcock

PROCEDURE

1. Identify a needle insertion site. Optimal insertion sites have a relatively flat surface with well-defined bony landmarks.
   a. Flat anterior medial surface of the proximal tibial shaft, 2 to 3 cm distal to the tibial tuberosity; this is a good site for almost all patients (Fig. 25-2*A, B*)
   b. Flat medial surface of the distal tibia, 2 to 3 cm proximal to the medial malleolus; this is a good site for older (>2 yr of age) children (Fig. 25-2*C*).
   c. Midline of the lower third of the femur, 3 to 4 cm above the external condyle; this site should only be used for small infants (Fig. 25-2*A, B*)

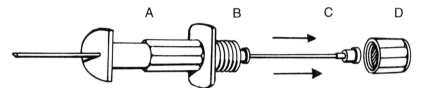

Figure 25–1. The Kormed/Jamshidi needle is most commonly used to obtain intraosseous access. Components include: *A*, Protective barrel to keep shaft from bending during insertion; *B*, Luer connector to secure infusion tubing; *C*, Stylet to prevent needle from filling with bone during insertion; *D*, Screw-on cap to protect Luer connector during insertion.

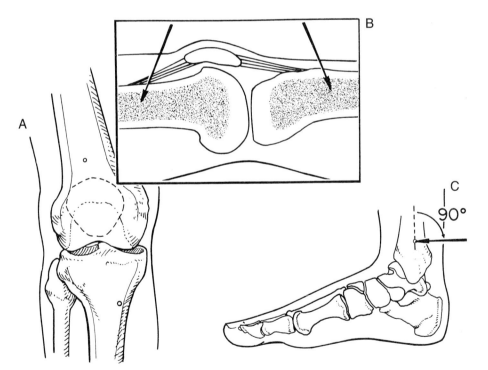

Figure 25–2. Optimal intraosseous insertion sites have a relatively flat surface. The anterior medial surface of the tibia is a good site in any age patient (*A, B*). The medial surface of the distal tibia can be safely used in children under 2 years of age (*C*). The lower third of the femur above the external condyle can be used safely only in small infants.

2. Prepare the selected site with Betadine.
3. If time permits (it usually does not), infiltrate the skin with 1% lidocaine.
4. Inspect the needle to ensure that the stylet is in place.
5. Insert the needle through the skin, then direct the needle at a slight 10- to 15-degree angle away from the perpendicular, directing the needle away from the adjacent underlying growth plate (Fig. 25-3).
6. Upon reaching bone, apply downward pressure using a rotary or twisting motion (Fig. 25-4).
7. Remove the stylet and confirm needle placement. If in place, attach IV tubing to needle Luer-Lok (Fig. 25-5).
8. Confirmation of intramedullary placement may be made by
   a. Release of resistance or "pop" after the needle passes through the bony cortex
   b. Aspiration of bloody bone marrow contents using a 20-cc syringe
      (**NOTE:** Aspirated marrow may not be readily apparent in small infants.)
   c. Rigid placement and positioning of the needle into the bone
   d. Free flowing of fluids into the marrow cavity
      (**NOTE:** Fluids rarely flow freely by gravity through an intraosseous needle. A pressure device or a stopcock and syringe may be needed to infuse fluids.)
9. If the procedure should fail, the next attempt should be made on the other extremity.

COMPLICATIONS

1. Osteomyelitis
2. Subcutaneous abscess
3. Fat or bone embolism
4. Injury to bone (induced fracture or epiphyseal damage)
5. Malposition or faulty insertion, either from failure to enter the bone or from passing the needle through the bone
6. Soft tissue or skin necrosis due to faulty insertion and drug administration and/or seepage into soft tissues
7. Injury to operator or assistant hand from placing hand under the extremity insertion site

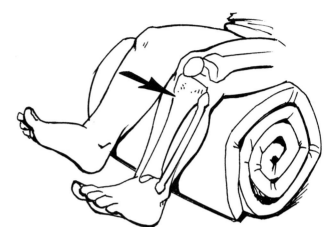

Figure 25–3. The needle is inserted through the skin and then directed 15 degrees below perpendicular away from the growth plate.

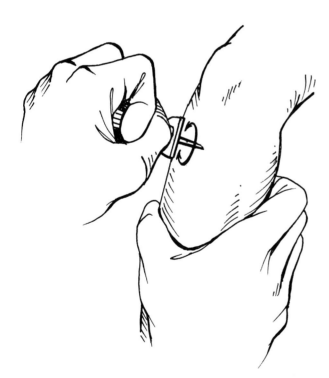

Figure 25–4. Upon reaching bone, apply downward pressure using a twisting motion.

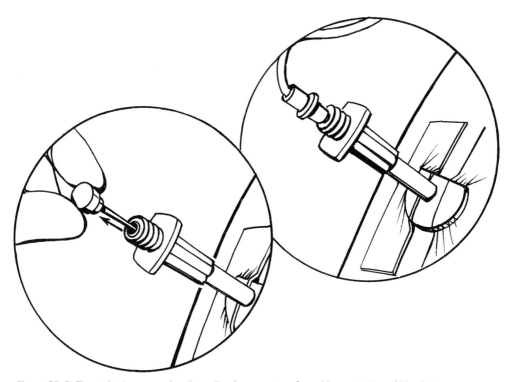

Figure 25–5. The stylet is removed and needle placement confirmed by aspiration of bloody bone marrow. If confirmed, attach intravenous tubing to the Luer connector. The fluid should infuse freely.

References

Chameides L, Hazinski MF (eds): *Textbook of Pediatric Advanced Life Support.* Dallas, American Heart Association, 1994, pp 5-5-5-7.

Glaeser PW, Losek JD: Intraosseus needles: New and improved. Pediatr Emerg Care 4:135-136, 1988.

Krug SE: Intraosseus infusion. In Blumer JB (ed): *A Practical Guide To Pediatric Intensive Care* (3rd ed). St Louis, Mosby-Year Book, 1990, pp 851-854.

Ruddy RM (ed): Illustrated techniques of pediatric emergency medicine. In Fleisher GR, Ludwig S (eds): *Textbook of Pediatric Emergency Medicine* (3rd ed). Baltimore, Williams & Wilkins, 1993, 1588-1589.

Spivey WH: Intraosseus infusion. In Roberts JR, Hedges JR (eds): *Clinical Procedures in Emergency Medicine* (2nd ed). Philadelphia, WB Saunders, 1991, pp 364-369.

Wagner MB, McCabe JB: A comparison of four techniques to establish intraosseus infusion. Pediatr Emerg Care 4:87-91, 1988.

CHAPTER 26

John T. Kanegaye

TOTALLY IMPLANTED VASCULAR ACCESS DEVICES

An increasingly large number of pediatric patients with chronic illnesses have undergone placement of subcutaneously implanted vascular access devices (e.g., MediPort, Port-a-Cath). Although they offer the advantage of long-term central venous access with minimal care needs, these devices are often unfamiliar to emergency care personnel. In addition, these devices are usually present in patients with limited alternatives for peripheral vascular access. As outlined here, the procedure for obtaining vascular access using these devices is relatively uncomplicated. However, minor variations in usage guidelines exist among institutions, particularly concerning the preferred long-term care of the device once accessed. Thus, it is prudent to be aware of the specific policies in effect at different institutions. In addition, the knowledgeable parent and patient can be a valuable resource for information regarding access and infusion.

INDICATIONS

1. Intravenous (IV) infusion of fluid or medication
2. Blood sampling

CONTRAINDICATIONS

1. Infection or decreased skin integrity over catheter port
2. Suspected catheter infection or occlusion (relative, as infusion of antibiotic or thrombolytic agent may be therapeutic)
3. Suspected catheter migration or malposition (relative, as contrast injection may be diagnostic)

EQUIPMENT

1. Huber's needle (noncoring) needle (3/4″, 1″, and 1-1/4″ depending on port and patient size) with extension tubing
2. Total parenteral nutrition (TPN) or central catheter dressing kit, *or* all of the following:
   a. Povidone-iodine swabs (3)
   b. Gauze sponges

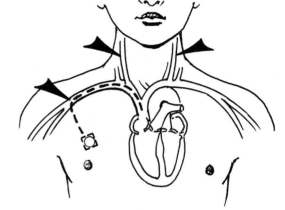

Figure 26–1. Identify the site of the implanted device by palpating the skin. Common sites of insertion are indicated by the arrows.

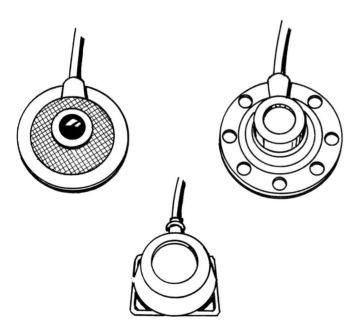

Figure 26–2. Several different types of implantable devices are currently in use.

    c. Sterile field

    d. Occlusive dressing

    e. Povidone-iodine ointment

3. Syringes for saline and heparin flush, blood sampling; discard as needed

4. Saline and heparin solution (100 U/cc)

5. Stopcock (optional)

6. Sterile gloves

7. Masks for patient and provider

PROCEDURE

1. Identify location of implanted device (Fig. 26-1).
   (**NOTE:** There are several different types and shapes presently in use.) (See Fig. 26-2)

2. Don mask and sterile gloves. Ideally, the patient and guardian should wear masks, if tolerated.

3. Prime stopcock, tubing, and Huber's needle with saline, leaving syringe attached (Fig. 26-3).

4. Prepare 10-cc syringe of saline flush (additional flush will be required if access is to be discontinued upon completion of blood draw) and heparin flush (500 U in 5 cc).

5. Cleanse skin over port with povidone-iodine solution, three times in gradually expanding concentric circles. Anesthetic infiltration is not generally performed, although prior application of eutectic mixture of local anesthetic (EMLA) may be considered in the nonurgent situation.

6. Palpate over the subcutaneous port and stabilize the port and the skin overlying the port with the fingers of the nondominant hand. Holding the primed Huber's needle-tubing assembly in the dominant hand, puncture the skin over the center of the port, penetrating the membrane to the entire depth of the port (Fig. 26-4).

7. Aspirate to confirm placement, and flush with saline to clear the line of previous heparin flush (some centers prefer to aspirate and discard at least 3 cc of dead space volume and blood to clear the line before initiating saline flush or infusion). At this point, fluid or medication may be infused directly into the Huber's needle-tubing assembly or through an interposed injection cap. Alternately, blood samples may be obtained from the tubing in the same manner as a central venous catheter (discarding 3 to 5 cc before withdrawal of desired samples). After blood draw, a second saline flush is recommended before initiating an infusion.

8. If the port is to remain accessed, povidone-iodide ointment is applied to the Huber's needle at the puncture site. If the extracutaneous portion of the Huber's needle does not sit flush against the skin, gauze sponges may be built up around the exposed needle for support. An occlusive dressing is applied over the Huber's needle-tubing assembly (Fig. 26-5).

9. To discontinue access, 10 cc of saline flush is infused followed by a heparin flush (500 U in 5 cc). The needle is withdrawn from the skin puncture site, and an adhesive strip bandage is applied (Fig. 26-6).

10. In event of difficulty withdrawing blood, the following maneuvers are recommended:

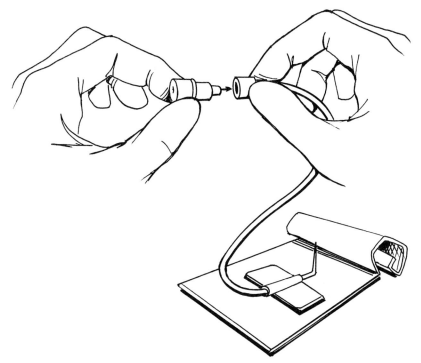

Figure 26–3. Assemble Huber needle, extension tubing, and cap. Flush with saline.

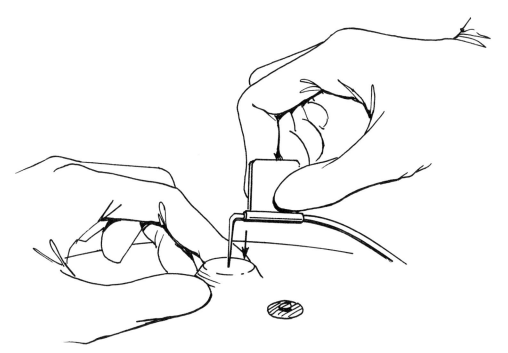

Figure 26–4. Stabilize the port with the fingers of the nondominant hand. Hold the primed Huber needle in the dominant hand and puncture the skin over the center of the port, and penetrate the full depth of the port.

CHAPTER 27

John T. Kanegaye

BROVIAC/HICKMAN ACCESS AND REPAIR

Although the use of subcutaneously tunneled catheters such as Broviac and Hickman catheters is similar to that of the familiar central venous monitoring catheter, various aspects of catheter care are different (particularly concerning discontinuation of access and aftercare). In addition, surprising variation in catheter care policies and equipment exists among institutions. Thus, it is prudent to be aware of specific policies at different institutions, which may vary from the guidelines given here. Very often, the experienced patient or parent may prove to be the most useful resource concerning the specific aspects of catheter care.

CATHETER ACCESS

INDICATIONS

1. Infusion of fluid or medication
2. Blood sampling

CONTRAINDICATIONS

1. Suspected catheter infection or occlusion (relative, may be therapeutic if antibiotic or thrombolytic infusion is planned)
2. Suspected catheter malposition/migration
3. Catheter rupture or fracture

EQUIPMENT

1. Syringes (5-12 cc)
2. Saline and heparin flush (usually 100 U/cc, although concentrations as low as 10 U/cc may be recommended for infants and younger children, depending on institutional policy)
3. Fluids and primed tubing, if needed for infusion
4. Heparin cap(s)
5. Stopcock (optional for sampling blood)

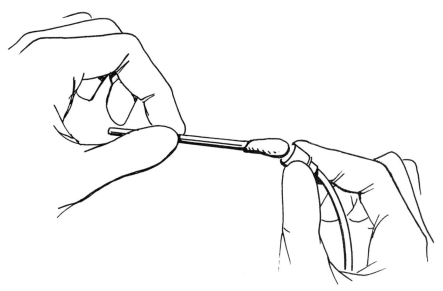

Figure 27–1. Scrub the injection cap with povidone-iodine solution or alcohol for 30 sec.

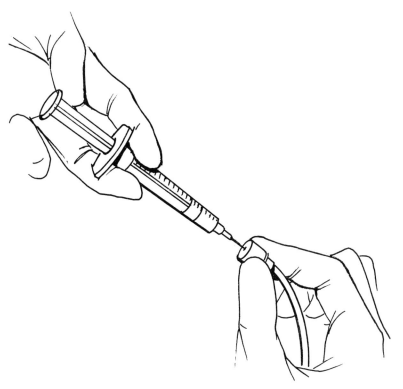

Figure 27–2. Puncture the cap with the needle and withdraw 3 to 5 cc of blood to clear the dead space.

PROCEDURE

1. Wash hands thoroughly with antiseptic solution. The use of nonsterile gloves is prudent, especially during blood sampling or infusion of blood products or chemotherapeutic agents.
2. Always clamp the catheter during removal of injection caps, changes of syringes and tubing, and at any other time that the distal end is left open to air. Most catheters are equipped with clamps that occlude the catheter at specially reinforced sites. If these are absent, the catheter may be clamped as described hereafter for catheter repair.
3. Blood sampling may be performed by one of several methods:
   a. For sampling by direct puncture of the injection cap, assemble needle, stopcock, and syringe. The stopcock permits the application of an additional syringe to the catheter without further manipulation. Scrub the injection cap with povidone-iodine solution or alcohol for 30 sec (Fig. 27-1). Puncture the injection cap with the needle-stopcock-syringe assembly and withdraw 3 to 5 cc of blood to clear dead space volume. (This volume, ordinarily discarded, may be used for culture if catheter infection is suspected.) (Fig. 27-2). Turn the stopcock off to change syringes, and withdraw the desired sample. Flush the lumen with saline. It may be prudent to aspirate a small amount of the dead space volume to evacuate air bubbles before flushing.
   b. Institutional policy may require removal of the injection cap with sampling directly from the catheter (Fig. 27-3). In this case, scrub the junction of the injection cap and catheter with povidone-iodine solution or alcohol for 30 sec. With the catheter clamped, remove the cap and similarly scrub the grooves at the distal end of the catheter. A stopcock may be used to avoid repetitive clamping of the catheter during changes of syringes.
4. Central venous infusion may be initiated directly or may follow blood sampling.
   a. For a single intravenous push, scrub the injection cap as in step 3(a). Puncture the cap with the needle and syringe containing the medication. Aspirate initially to confirm intravenous catheter placement, and proceed with the injection in the manner recommended for the specific medication. Flush with saline and then with heparin solution. Note that drugs prepared in small volumes or high concentrations may be retained in significant amounts within the dead space of the catheter, and an inadvertent rapid bolus may result during saline flush despite slow injection of the medication itself.

   or
   b. For prolonged infusion, the injection cap may be scrubbed as in 3(a) and the catheter accessed with direct puncture of the cap by needle attached to the infusion tubing.

   or
   c. Alternately, the infusion tubing may be connected directly to the distal end of the catheter after removal of the injection cap, using the technique described in 3(c).
5. In the event of difficulty withdrawing blood, the following maneuvers are recommended:
   a. Examine the course of the catheter for kinking or undetected clamp.
   b. Reposition the patient (have him or her sit up, turn to sides, vary position of arms, assume Trendelenburg position, attempt Valsalva maneuver).
   c. Flush additional saline prior to resuming attempts at aspiration of blood.
   d. Attempt aspiration of blood sample with a smaller syringe.

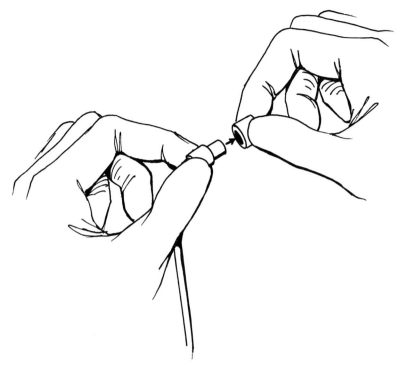

Figure 27–3. Institutional policy may require removal of the injection cap. Be sure to clamp the catheter before this is removed.

    e. If sampling through heparin cap, consider removal of cap with sampling directly from the catheter.

6. The possibility of catheter malposition, or occlusion, may need to be considered. If blood withdrawal or infusion is not possible, consider evaluating for occlusion or malposition as follows:

    a. Radiograph chest to confirm location.

    b. A contrast study may further elucidate the nature of the occlusion. Specialty consultation is highly recommended before proceeding with this or other interventions.

    c. Thrombolytic therapy may be attempted with 1 to 2 ml of urokinase (2500 to 5000 U/ml) injected into the occluded catheter, and repeated in 1 hour if aspiration remains impossible. Low-dose urokinase infusion may be required for persistent occlusion (200 U/kg/hr over 24 hr). Specialty consultation is recommended.

COMPLICATIONS

1. Introduction of infection
2. Air embolus or loss of blood during injection or undetected disconnection of tubing
3. Catheter occlusion due to mechanical factors or inadequate heparinization
4. Infusion into pleural or mediastinal space owing to undetected catheter malposition or migration
5. Systemic heparinization

REPAIR OF CATHETER

NOTE: This procedure is described in detail in manuals sealed within commercially available repair kits. However, the procedure is best performed with advance knowledge of the general approach to repair outlined here.

EQUIPMENT

1. Repair kit appropriate to the number and diameter of lumens at the proposed site of repair
2. Scalpel
3. Sterile syringes and needles
4. Normal saline and heparin solution
5. Povidone-iodine swabs
6. Sterile gloves and drapes (the use of masks, cap, and sterile gown may further minimize the risk of contamination)
7. Clamp: Many types of clamps are available for this purpose. The desired features of any device used to occlude a catheter include surfaces without ridges or teeth such as are present on many surgical clamps; jaws that close in a controlled fashion to prevent crushing of the catheter; and, if possible, surfaces that are constructed of plastic or shod with rubber.
8. Tongue blade and tape

PROCEDURE

1. Atraumatically clamp the catheter proximal to the site of rupture, far enough from the rupture to allow the clamp to be isolated by sterile drapes. The catheter's own clamp and reinforced segment are preferred for this purpose but are often not available or intact proximal to the rupture. If a clamp is applied to the double-lumen portion of a catheter, the jaws of the clamp should be oriented parallel to the septum separating the two lumens (Fig. 27–4). Ideally, this maneuver will have been performed by the patient prior to presentation.
2. If a concentrated dextrose solution ($\geq$10%) had been infusing prior to rupture, it is prudent to monitor the patient for hypoglycemia.
3. Position the patient in the supine position. A mask may be worn by the patient and any others present, if tolerated.
4. Open the repair kit in a sterile manner on a sterile towel. Don mask, sterile gloves, and gown.
5. While an assistant holds the distal end of the catheter away from the patient's body, paint the exposed length of the catheter three times with povidone-iodine solution. (This step may be performed prior to donning sterile gloves.)
6. With the distal end of the ruptured lumen still suspended, place drapes on patient's chest to isolate the now-sterile repair site from the patient's skin and from unscrubbed regions of the catheter.
7. Determine the site of repair by identifying a location between the proximal clamp and the rupture that provides at least 2 to 3 cm of surrounding intact catheter. Sharply divide the catheter at this site, and discard the damaged distal portion (Fig. 27–5).

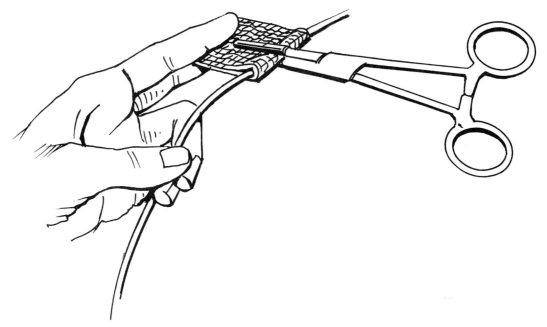

Figure 27–4. Atraumatically clamp the catheter using the catheter's own clamp and reinforced segment. If these are not available, use a guarded tubing clamp and cover the catheter with gauze to protect the lumen.

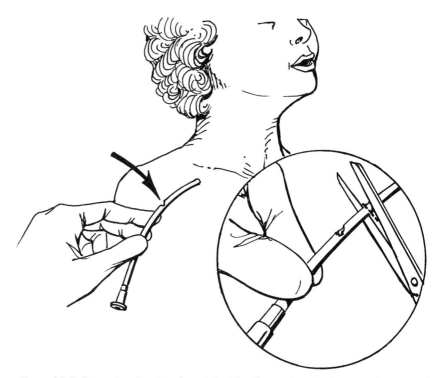

Figure 27–5. Determine the site of repair by identifying a location between the proximal clamp and the rupture that gives at least 2 cm of intact catheter. Sharply divide the catheter at this point and discard the damaged distal portion.

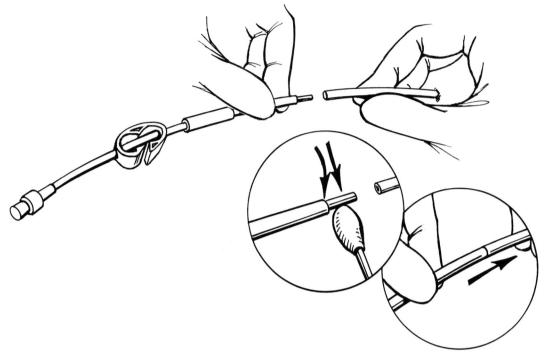

Figure 27–6. Prepare the replacement portion by applying adhesive to the metal adapter, taking great care to avoid introducing the adhesive into the lumen. Insert the adapter into the portion of the incised catheter that is inserted into the patient.

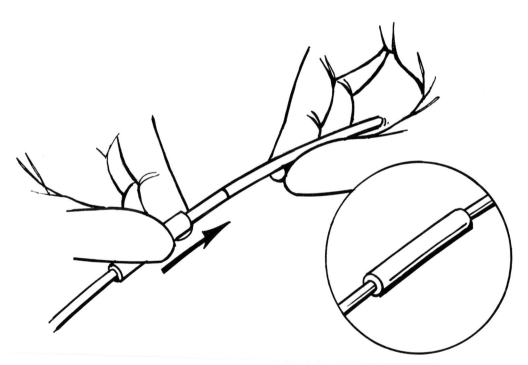

Figure 27–7. Push the catheter ends together and slide the plastic sleeve over the repair site. Introduce adhesive under the sleeve and roll between fingers to evenly distribute adhesive.

8. Apply adhesive to the metal adapter of the replacement tubing, taking care to avoid occluding its lumen. Insert the adapter into the lumen of the proximal portion of the incised catheter (Fig. 27-6). Slide the plastic sleeve provided with the replacement tubing over the repair site (Fig. 27-7). Introduce adhesive under the sleeve and roll between fingers to distribute evenly.
9. Attach saline-filled syringe to the newly repaired catheter. Release the proximal clamp and aspirate blood to evacuate air in dead space and to confirm catheter patency. Flush with saline, cap the catheter, and flush with heparin. If provided, close catheter clamp(s) at appropriate reinforced segment.
10. Splint the repair site with tongue blade and tape.

COMPLICATIONS

1. Introduction of infection
2. Inadvertent injection of air or intraluminal thrombus
3. Inability to complete repair owing to occlusion of lumen, unavailability of appropriate repair kit, or insufficient length of intact extracutaneous catheter

References

Alexander HR. Vascular access and other specialized techniques of drug delivery. In Devita VT, Hellman S, Rosenberg SA (eds): *Cancer: Principles and Practice of Oncology* (4th ed). Philadelphia, JB Lippincott, 1989, pp 556-564.

Bagnall H, Gomperts E, Atkinson J. Continuous infusion of low dose urokinase in the treatment of central venous catheter thrombosis in infants and children. Pediatrics 83:963-966, 1989.

Marcoux C, Fisher S, Wong D. Central venous access devices in children. Pediatr Nurs 16:123-133, 1990.

Raaf JH. Results from use of 826 vascular access devices in cancer patients. Cancer 55:1312-1321, 1985.

Winthrop AL, Wesson DE. Urokinase in the treatment of occluded central venous catheters in children. J Pediatr Surg 19:536-538, 1984.

SECTION 4

DIAGNOSTIC AND THERAPEUTIC PROCEDURES

CHAPTER 28

Michele Walsh-Sukys

THORACENTESIS

INDICATIONS

1. Obtain fluid for diagnostic evaluation.
2. To relieve respiratory compromise, drain fluid that is unlikely to reaccumulate.
3. Emergently evacuate tension pneumothorax until a tube thoracostomy can be placed.
4. Electively evacuate pneumothorax when the air is unlikely to reaccumulate (such as following an intrathoracic procedure).

CONTRAINDICATIONS

None

EQUIPMENT

1. Sterile gloves
2. Sterile drapes
3. Betadine
4. Local anesthetic
5. 22-g angiocatheter
6. T connector
7. 3-way stopcock
8. Syringe

TECHNIQUE

1. Position the patient:
   a. For neonates and mechanically ventilated patients, the supine position with a towel placed underneath the hemithorax to elevate the chest wall above the bed sheets is preferred.
   b. For older children, the seated position with arms folded on a bedside table and the head resting on the arms may be preferred.
2. Prepare the skin surface with Betadine solution.
3. Locate the fourth intercostal space in the mid-axillary line (the level of the nipple), and place sterile drapes over the area.

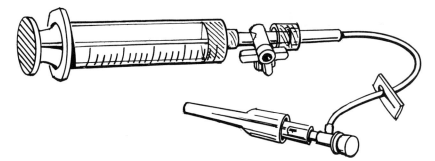

Figure 28–1. Assembly of equipment typically used in thoracentesis. An angiocath with trochar is connected to a T connector, stopcock, and then syringe.

4. Connect the angiocatheter with trochar in place to the T connector, stopcock, and syringe (Fig. 28–1).
5. Insert the angiocatheter over the superior border of the rib in the mid-axillary line, and direct it anteriorly and superiorly toward the apex of the lung to evacuate air. If fluid is being removed, then one will enter in the posterior-axillary line and direct the catheter inferiorly and posteriorly. Insert until a "pop" is felt, generally about 1 to 2 cm (Fig. 28–2).
6. If the thoracentesis is for air, turn the stopcock to the open position and withdraw air into the syringe. If the syringe fills completely, close the stopcock and empty the syringe and then repeat until all air is evacuated. One may wish to leave the angiocatheter in place until certain that no air will reaccumulate. If this is the case, then the metal trochar must be removed to prevent laceration

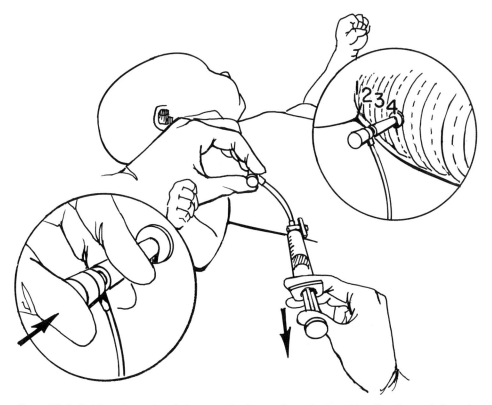

Figure 28–2. Stabilize the angiocath between the fingers. Insert in the mid-axillary line and direct the needle in the direction of the fluid or air to be sampled. (See text for further details.)

of the lung. One must check for air reaccumulation every 10 min by applying negative pressure to the syringe. If evidence of air reaccumulation is found, then a thoracostomy tube should be inserted.

7. If the thoracentesis is for fluid, turn the stopcock to the open position and withdraw fluid into the syringe.

Alternative Technique for Fluid Collection

Recently in adults an alternative technique has been described for diagnostic thoracentesis. Previous steps 1 through 3 are followed. A Vacutainer (Becton-Dickinson) blood collection device is then used. The prepared skin is penetrated with a needle, and suction is applied to the needle while in the soft tissue. The needle is then advanced into the pleural space and fluid is collected directly into the appropriate tube. The procedure is safe, effective, and resulted in fewer pneumothoraces than the conventional technique. Patients generally report the procedure to be less painful than the standard technique.

Laboratory Analysis of Fluid

The first step in evaluation is to distinguish transudates from exudates. Transudates develop from elevated capillary hydrostatic pressure or from decreased colloid osmotic pressure. Common causes include congestive heart failure, cirrhosis, nephrotic syndrome, and constrictive pericarditis. Exudates are caused by obstruction of the lymphatic vessels or altered permeability of the pleural vessels. Common causes include malignancy, infection, or inflammatory diseases. In pediatric patients some series have suggested that infection accounts for 85% of all effusions, thus most will be exudates, and all will require bacteriologic evaluation. Traditionally this has been approached by sending all specimens for a panel of studies: culture, gram's stain, complete cell count, protein, lactic dehydrogenase (LDH), glucose, amylase, and pH. Exudates have at least one of the following characteristics (and transudates have none): (1) pleural fluid protein to serum protein ratio of >0.5, (2) pleural fluid LDH to serum ratio >0.6, and 3) pleural fluid LDH greater than two-thirds the upper limit of normal for serum LDH. Peterman and Speicher recommend a two-stage approach in adults as a more cost-effective method for evaluating effusions:

1. Identify transudates by measuring serum and pleural fluid protein and LDH. Specimens identified as transudates would need no further testing.
2. All other specimens would be sent for a full panel of tests.

COMPLICATIONS

1. Pneumothorax
2. Infection
3. Laceration of the intercostal artery or vein. Since the neurovascular bundle lies on the underneath side of the rib, misplacement of the needle may lacerate a blood vessel. If this occurs surgical correction may be necessary. Laceration can be avoided by sliding the needle over the superior aspect of the rib when introducing it.

4. Puncture of the lung parenchyma. If the needle is advanced too far it may pierce the lung parenchyma. This may be avoided by halting insertion after a "pop" is felt. If blood is obtained after the needle has been inserted, it should be assumed that a laceration of the lung has occurred. Promptly remove the needle. Most lacerations seal spontaneously. If fluid accumulation is revealed by radiograph, surgical exploration is needed.

5. Puncture of the heart. If the needle is advanced too far, and directed medially rather than toward the apex, the heart may be pierced. This may be detected when a large volume of free flowing blood is returned. If the needle is withdrawn promptly, the puncture usually seals immediately. If fluid accumulation is revealed by radiograph, surgical exploration is needed.

6. Laceration of intra-abdominal organs. Needles inadvertently inserted below the diaphragm may lacerate solid organs. Splenic laceration may require surgical repair to ensure adequate hemostasis.

References

Azedo I, Sarbeji M, LeBourgeois M, et al. Diagnostic evaluation of pleural effusion in children. Report of 59 cases. Pediatrie Bucutr 45:807–812, 1990.

Bartter T, Mayo PD, Pratter MR, et al. Lower risk and higher yield for thoracentesis when performed by experienced operators. Chest 103:1873–1876, 1993.

Collins TR, Sahn SA. Thoracentesis: Clinical value, complications, technical problems, and patient experience. Chest 91:817–822, 1987.

Govig B, Balton M. Simplified bedside thoracentesis (letter). Ann Intern Med 120:695–696, 1994.

Grogan DR, Irwin RS, Channick R, et al. Complications associated with thoracentesis: A prospective, randomized study of three different methods. Arch Inter Med 150:873–877, 1990.

Light RW, MacGregor MI, Luchsinger PC, et al. The diagnostic separation of transudates and exudates. Ann Intern Med 77:507–513, 1972.

Peterman TA, Speicher CE. Evaluating pleural effusions. A two stage laboratory approach. JAMA 252:1051–1053, 1984.

Sokolowski JW Jr, Burgher LW, Jones FL Jr, et al. Guidelines for thoracentesis and needle biopsy of the pleura. A position paper of the ATS board of directors. Am Rev Respir Dis 140:257–258, 1989.

CHAPTER 29

Michele Walsh-Sukys

THORACOSTOMY

INDICATIONS

1. Prolonged drainage of air or fluid from the chest
2. Drainage of empyema
3. Drainage of hemothorax
4. Definitive treatment of tension pneumothorax
5. Occasionally used as route to deliver anesthetic or chemotherapeutic agents to pleural space

CONTRAINDICATIONS

1. Systemic heparinization (relative)

EQUIPMENT

1. Sterile gloves
2. Sterile drapes
3. Betadine
4. Local anesthetic
5. Thoracostomy tube, size appropriate to patient and material to be drained (see Appendix A)
6. Scalpel
7. Kelly clamp
8. Suture
9. Occlusive dressing

TECHNIQUE

1. If time permits, the skin, subcutaneous tissue, and rib margins should be anesthetized with lidocaine. Older children and adults rate thoracostomy among the most painful procedures. Therefore, an intravenous (IV) opiate analgesic should be considered (see Chapter 3).
2. Prepare the skin with Betadine, and drape in a sterile manner.
3. Make a 1-cm incision through the skin and subcutaneous tissue along the vertical margin of the fifth or sixth rib in the anterior axillary line. Some authors have recommended placing chest tubes in the mid-clavicular line as

these may be most effective in removing anterior pockets of air in a supine patient. However, destruction of breast tissue may occur with this approach, leading to a cosmetically unacceptable result in the future. Therefore, we recommend that this approach be avoided.

4. Insert a closed Kelly clamp through the incision, track up two interspaces, and, over the superior aspect of the rib, push through the intercostal muscle and pleura into the pleural space. Spread the clamp to enlarge the opening to admit the chest tube (Fig. 29-1).

5. If the tube is being placed to drain air, and since air rises anteriorly in a supine patient, one wishes to direct the tube anteriorly and superiorly (Fig. 29-2). Turning the Kelly clamp so that the curve is facing up will help direct the thoracostomy tube to the optimal location. Slide the tube over the superior aspect of the clamp into position. The optimal insertion length can be estimated by laying the tube on the chest wall and marking the position where the tube should emerge from the skin with a silk tie. Allow 2 to 3 cm for tunneling the tube.

6. If the tube is being placed to drain fluid, then the optimal placement is inferiorly and posteriorly (Fig. 29-2).

7. Connect the tube either to a closed pleural drainage device (Fig. 29-2) or to a Heimlich valve (Fig. 29-3).

8. Many chest tubes will come supplied with a trochar. In most instances it is desirable to place the chest tube using the Kelly clamp alone, rather than the trochar, because trochars have been associated with an increased frequency of lung laceration. If a trochar is used, the tip must be partially withdrawn so that its tip is well within the chest tube.

9. Alternative technique: In neonates an alternative technique has been described in which the tip of the Kelly clamp is placed in the most distal hole of the chest tube and inserted with the curve of the clamp directed toward the desired location. Both the clamp and the tube are inserted together, and then the clamp is opened and withdrawn.

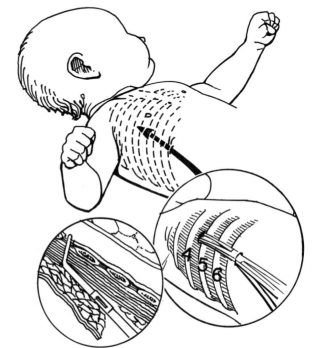

Figure 29–1. Make a 1-cm incision through the skin and subcutaneous tissue along the superior rib margin in the anterior axillary line. Insert a closed Kelly clamp, track up two interspaces, and apply pressure until the pleura is breached. Open the clamp to enlarge the opening and admit the chest tube.

10. Suture the tube in place. Some surgeons prefer to create a purse string tie around the chest tube to decrease the likelihood of its dislodging. However, this suturing technique creates a scar that may be cosmetically unacceptable. Therefore, closing the wound on either side of the chest tube with two interrupted stitches may be preferable. A self-retaining suture may be placed in the skin and then the chest tube secured with this suture (see Fig. 23-5).

11. A very small air-tight dressing should be placed over the wound. Transparent dressings are sometimes used for this; however, the majority of these dressings are meant to enhance wound healing by permitting air entry, and thus may not be appropriate. It is quite important that the dressing be small; otherwise the entire chest wall in a small infant may be splinted with the dressing, further compromising ventilation.

12. Assess for correct chest tube placement with an anterior and lateral view of the chest. Chest tubes that cross or impinge on the mediastinum must be pulled back to avoid compromising cardiac output by aortic compression.

Pigtail (Minithoracostomy) Technique

1. Investigators have recently reported a new technique which is potentially less traumatic than traditional thoracostomy placement. In these techniques smaller catheters are inserted over guidewires using a modification of Seldinger's technique.

2. A needle is introduced into the pleural space. A guidewire is advanced into the needle. The needle is removed, while the wire is carefully held stationary.

3. To enlarge the puncture site, a dilator is advanced over the wire, penetrating about 1 in into the pleural space. The dilator is then removed.

4. The pigtail catheter is then advanced over the wire, and the wire withdrawn. The catheter is connected to a closed pleural drainage system using an adapter. This newer technique has not been evaluated in large numbers of patients, but may prove beneficial in selected settings.

COMPLICATIONS

1. Improper position
   a. If the pleural space is not entered, a tube can be placed in subcutaneous tissue resulting in therapeutic delays. This placement can be detected by palpating the chest wall and feeling the tube.
   b. A tube that is inserted too far may impinge on mediastinal structures and can cause obstruction of the aorta or lead to vascular erosion.
2. Hemorrhage
   a. Laceration of the intercostal artery or vein. Because the neurovascular bundle lies on the underneath side of the rib, misplacement of the needle may cause laceration of a blood vessel. If this occurs, surgical correction may be necessary. Laceration can be avoided by sliding the tube over the superior aspect of the rib when introducing it.
   b. Laceration of the pulmonary artery, vein, or aorta by trochar or by tube (the tube should be introduced gently, and never forced if resistance is met)
   c. Laceration of the heart
3. Puncture of the lung parenchyma: If the tube or trochar are advanced too far

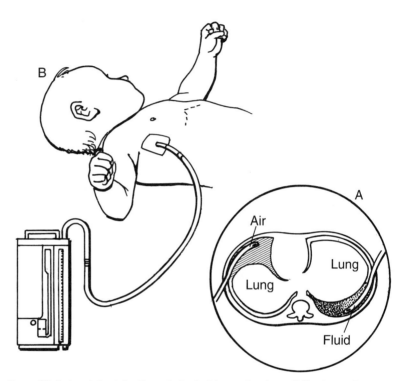

Figure 29–2. Insert the tube through the incision and, using a Kelly clamp, direct the tube into position. The tube should be placed anteriorly, to remove air, and posteriorly, to remove fluid. The tube is then connected to a closed device that either has an underwater seal or is on negative pressure.

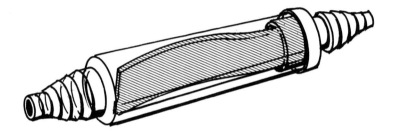

Figure 29–3. If suction or underwater seal is unavailable, a Heimlich valve, which provides for one-way flow of air out of the chest, may be effectively used. This is most frequently used during transport.

they may pierce the lung parenchyma. This may be avoided by halting insertion after a "pop" is felt. If blood is obtained after the tube has been inserted, it should be assumed that a laceration of the lung has occurred. Most lacerations will seal spontaneously. If fluid accumulation is revealed by radiograph, surgical exploration is usually required.

4. Laceration of intra-abdominal organs. Tubes that are inadvertently inserted below the diaphragm may lacerate solid organs including the liver, spleen, or diaphraghm. Hepatic or splenic laceration may require surgical repair to adequately ensure hemostasis.

5. Infection: Infection at the chest tube site is a common complication. Careful skin preparation and dressing changes may lessen its frequency.

6. Neurologic injury: Traumatic injury of the intercostal nerve is a well-described complication of thoracostomy placement. Acute injury to the phrenic nerve with resultant diaphragmatic paralysis and diaphragmatic eventration also have been described.

7. Pneumothorax

8. Chylothorax may occur following thoracostomy placement if the thoracic duct is injured. The chances of this may be minimized by ensuring that the tube does not impinge on the mediastinum.

References

Allen RW, Jung Al, Lester PD. Effectiveness of chest tube evacuation of pneumothoraces in neonates. J Pediatr 99:629–633, 1981.

Banagle RC, Outerbridge EW, Aranda JV. Lung perforation: A complication of chest tube insertion in neonatal pneumothorax. J Pediatr 94:973–975, 1979.

Gilmartin JJ, Wright AJ, Gibson GJ. Effects of pneumothorax or pleural effusion on pulmonary function. Thorax 40:60–66, 1985.

Gooding C, Kerlan R Jr, Brasch R. Partial aortic obstruction produced by a thoracostomy tube. J Pediatr 98:471–473, 1981.

Guyton SW, Paull DL, Anderson RP. Introducer insertion of mini-thoracostomy tubes. Am J Surg 155:693–696, 1988.

Heimlich HJ. Valve drainage of the pleural cavity. Dis Chest 53:282–285, 1968.

Jung A, Minton S, Roan Y. Pulmonary hemorrhage after chest tube placement for pneumothorax in neonates. Clin Pediatr 19:624–626, 1980.

Jung AL, Nelson J, Jenkins MB, et al. Clinical evaluation of a new chest tube used in neonates. Clin Pediatr 30:85–87, 1991.

Kumar SP, Bellik J. Chylothorax—a complication of chest tube placement. Crit Care Med 12:411–415, 1984.

Lackey DA, Urainski CT, Taber P. The management of tension pneumothorax in the neonate using the Heimlich flutter valve. J Pediatr 84:438–441, 1974.

Lawless S, Orr R, Killian A, et al. New pigtail catheter for pleural drainage in pediatric patients. Crit Care Med 17:173–175, 1989.

Mandansky DL, Lawson EE, Chernick V, et al. Pneumothorax and other forms of air leak in newborns. Am Rev Respir Dis 120:729–732, 1979.

Marinelli P, Ortiz A, Alden ER. Acquired eventration of the diaphragm: A complication of chest tube placement in neonatal pneumothorax. Pediatr 67:552–553, 1981.

Mehrabani D, Kopelman AE. Chest tube insertion: A simplified technique. Pediatrics 83:784–785, 1989.

Moessinger AC, Driscoll JM, Wigger HJ. High incidence of lung perforation by chest tubes in neonatal pneumothorax. J Pediatr 92:635–637, 1978.

Ogata ES, Gregory GA, Kitterman JA, et al. Pneumothorax in the respiratory distress syndrome: Incidence, effects on vital signs, blood gases and pH. Pediatrics 58:177–184, 1976.

Phillips A, Rowe J, Raye J: Acute diaphragmatic paralysis after chest tube placement in the neonate. AJR 136:824–825, 1981.

Sacks LM. Lung perforation by chest tubes. J Pediatr 94:341, 1979.

Wilson AJ, Krous HF. Lung perforation during chest tube placement in the stiff lung syndrome. J Pediatr Surg 9:213–215, 1974.

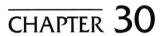

CHAPTER 30

Brenda R. Hook

PERICARDIOCENTESIS

INDICATIONS

1. Air, blood, or other fluid within the pericardial space causing symptoms of cardiovascular compromise
2. An acutely decompensating patient with muffled or absent heart sounds, decreased pulse pressure, and/or identification of air in the pericardial sac

CONTRAINDICATIONS

None

EQUIPMENT

1. Sterile drapes and gloves
2. Betadine solution
3. Angiocatheter suitable to size of patient
4. 3-way stopcock
5. Intravenous fluid (IVF) tubing connectors (T connectors)
6. 5-cc or 10-cc Luer-Lok syringe
7. Occlusive dressing

TECHNIQUE

1. Ensure patient is on a dynamic cardiorespiratory monitor.
2. Select an angiocatheter of an appropriate length for the size of the patient. A 20-gauge angiocatheter is appropriate for most term newborns, a 2.5-in 18-gauge angiocatheter will suffice for younger children, and a 3.5-in long pericardial or spinal needle for adolescents.
3. Prepare the angiocatheter by attaching the T connector to the needle hub and attaching this apparatus to the 3-way stopcock. The syringe should be attached to the stopcock so air or fluid may be withdrawn from the pericardial sac and then flushed out the third port of the stopcock.
4. Prepare the sub-xiphoid area with Betadine and surround with sterile drapes.
5. Wearing sterile gloves, isolate the xiphoid process with one hand. At about 1 cm below the xiphoid process insert the angiocatheter at about a 20- to 30-degree angle to the skin (Fig. 30–1). Slowly advance the angiocatheter while

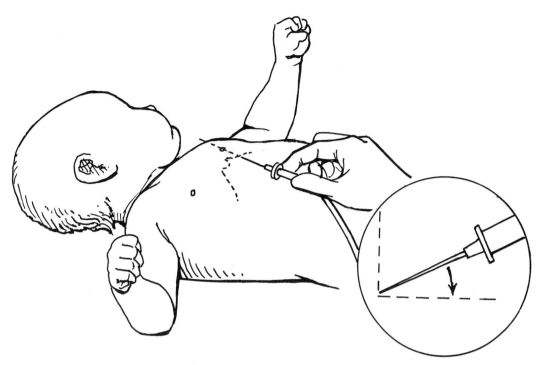

Figure 30–1. To perform a pericardiocentesis, attach a T connector, 3-way stopcock, and syringe to an angiocath. Insert the needle at a 20- to 30-degree angle under the xiphoid process, while continuously drawing back on the syringe. Aim toward the left shoulder.

monitoring the patient's cardiac rhythm, aiming at the tip of the left shoulder. Be careful to go under the xiphoid process but not too deep. In neonates, transillumination of the pericardial sac with a high-intensity fiberoptic light may be helpful.

6. Continue to advance slowly while applying light negative pressure with the syringe. If a cardiac rhythm disturbance is noted, withdraw the needle 1 to 2 cm. After the air or fluid returns in the T connector, *stop* advancing the catheter and aspirate a small amount to confirm positioning (Fig. 30-2).

7. Remove the T connector from the angiocatheter and rapidly hold your finger over the needle hub. Advance the catheter portion farther into the pericardial space and remove the needle. Reattach the T connector and resume aspiration of the air or fluid. Any fluid aspirated should be sent for cell count, chemistry, and culture.

8. Tape or suture the angiocatheter in place. Obtain a chest radiograph to confirm positioning and effect of procedure.

9. If reaccumulation occurs, surgery consultation should be obtained for placement of a pericardial tube.

COMPLICATIONS

1. Laceration of the heart wall—the most common and lethal complication. The needle should be withdrawn slightly if blood is aspirated. The best way to avoid laceration is to advance slowly and remove the needle before aspiration of a large amount of pericardial air or fluid. The air or fluid will act as a cushion to

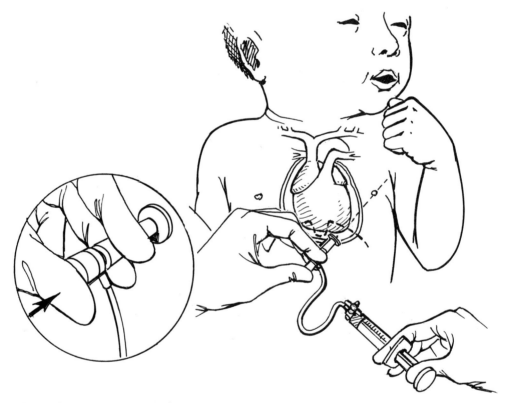

Figure 30–2. Halt the advance of the needle when air or fluid is returned or if a cardiac rhythm disturbance occurs.

protect the heart wall from the needle until the catheter is advanced and the needle removed.

2. Malfunction of the angiocatheter after placement—common. In an acutely decompensated patient, the angiocatheter should simply be replaced using the technique described, or over a wire in a stabilized patient. Surgical consultation should be obtained for placement of a pericardial tube.

3. Risk of infection is a problem with any indwelling catheter. Meticulous attention to sterile technique and catheter removal, or replacement after 72 hours, will help decrease the incidence of pericarditis.

4. Pneumothorax

5. Pneumopericardium

6. Cardiac rhythm disturbances

References

Cabatu EE, Brown EG: Thoracic transillumination: Aid in the diagnosis and treatment of pneumopericardium. Pediatrics 64:958-960, 1979.

Emery RW, Foker J, Thompson TR: Neonatal pneumopericardium: A surgical emergency. Ann Thorac Surg 37:128-132, 1984.

Emery RW, Lindsay WG, Nicoloff DM: Placement of pericardial drainage tube for the treatment of pneumopericardium in the neonate. Ann Thorac Surg 26:84-87, 1978.

Lawson EE, Gould JB, Taeusch HW: Neonatal pneumopericardium: Current management. J Pediatr Surg 15:181-185, 1980.

Pomerance JJ, Weller MH, Richardson CJ et al: Pneumopericardium complicating respiratory distress syndrome: Role of conservative management. J Pediatr 84:883-885, 1974.

Reppert SM, Ment LR, Todres ID: Treatment of pneumopericardium in the newborn infant. J Pediatr 90:115-118, 1977.

CHAPTER 31

John T. Kanegaye

PARACENTESIS

INDICATIONS

1. Sampling of peritoneal fluid for evaluation of ascites
2. Relief of respiratory compromise caused by accumulation of peritoneal fluid
3. Evaluation for the presence of hemoperitoneum is not considered an appropriate indication for paracentesis, as other modalities are preferable.

CONTRAINDICATIONS

1. Bleeding diathesis or thrombocytopenia (relative)
2. Infection overlying proposed site of puncture
3. Presence of known adhesions or previous surgical procedure(s) in the region of the proposed puncture site
4. Organomegaly or abdominal mass in the region of the proposed puncture site
5. Severe bowel distention
6. Inability to empty the patient's bladder
7. Highly agitated or uncooperative patient
8. Pregnancy (relative)
9. Presence of another abdominal condition necessitating laparotomy

EQUIPMENT

1. Supplies for asepsis
   a. Sterile drapes
   b. Sterile gloves
   c. Prep solution (generally povidone-iodine)
   d. Shave kit for the hirsute patient
2. Lidocaine (1% with epinephrine) for local infiltration
3. Sterile syringes
   a. 1- to 3-ml for infiltration of anesthetic
   b. 10-ml for aspiration (larger sizes for relief of abdominal distention)
4. Sterile needles
   a. 25-gauge for local infiltration
   b. 18- to 22-gauge spinal needle for aspiration,
   or

c. Over-the-needle intravenous (IV) catheter (18- to 22-gauge),

or

d. Through-the-needle IV catheter (18- to 20-gauge)

5. Stopcock and/or short IV connecting tubing (optional adjuncts permitting changes of syringes and giving leeway for motion in the uncooperative patient)

6. Specimen collection tubes

7. Collection bottle for large-volume paracentesis (plastic tubing and bags used in blood banking provide a closed system convenient for this purpose)

8. Sterile gauze sponges and dressing supplies

PROCEDURE

1. Prepare the patient for the procedure.
   a. Consider correction of significant coagulopathy or thrombocytopenia.
   b. Have the patient empty his or her bladder, or insert a Foley catheter.
   c. Consider establishing venous access to correct potential intravascular volume depletion precipitated by removal of large amounts of peritoneal fluid.
2. Choose the puncture site based on clinical findings and contraindications, as outlined earlier. Almost any surface of the abdominal wall is available for this procedure; however, the right and left lower quadrants lateral to the rectus muscles are convenient locations, minimizing the risk of perforation of the epigastric arteries or an enlarged liver or spleen. The midline of the abdomen below the umbilicus is also favorable, as there is decreased vascularity in this region. If the presence or localization of the peritoneal fluid collection is in doubt, consider the use of ultrasound guidance.
3. Position the patient appropriately for the chosen puncture site.
   a. For lower-quadrant puncture, turning the supine patient toward the side of the puncture will allow the bowel to float upward with dependent accumulation of peritoneal fluid (Fig. 31–1).
   b. For midline puncture, various positions will facilitate fluid collection including lateral decubitus, semirecumbent, sitting, and knee-chest (Fig. 31–2).
4. Don sterile gloves (and mask).
5. Paint the skin of the abdominal wall three times with a solution of povidone-iodine, starting from the puncture site and expanding outward in a concentric fashion.
6. Apply sterile drapes.
7. Create a subcutaneous wheal of lidocaine at the proposed puncture site.

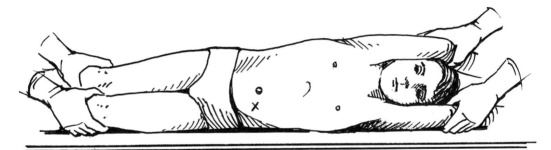

Figure 31–1. Various positions are available in which to safely perform paracentesis. The lower quadrants lateral to the abdomen are avascular and quite safe. The patient is placed supine and rolled toward the side of the puncture, which allows the bowel to float upward and out of the way. The puncture site is indicated with an X.

8. Puncture the abdominal wall with a styletted spinal needle, or needle and syringe assembly (Fig. 31-3). Advancing the needle in a Z-track manner or at an angle away from the perpendicular may minimize subsequent leakage of fluid. Entry into the peritoneal cavity is indicated by a distinct decrease in resistance (often appreciated as a "pop") and is confirmed by aspiration of fluid. If a flexible catheter is used, it is advanced over (or through) the needle into the peritoneal cavity. Vascular catheters are particularly useful in preventing inadvertent trauma if one anticipates patient movement, the need to manipulate the catheter or patient, or the aspiration of a large volume of fluid.

9. Obtain the desired sample of peritoneal fluid for laboratory studies. For large-volume paracentesis, multiple changes of syringes are facilitated by the use of a stopcock, with an optional intervening length of infusion tubing. Alternatively, a longer length of infusion tubing leading to a large collection bottle or bag may be incorporated into the collection system by means of a 3-way stopcock. Although paracentesis of 1000 cc/24 hr is considered safe in adults, guidelines for volume of pediatric paracentesis are not widely established. In the absence of sound scientific findings, it is prudent to limit pediatric paracentesis to a comparable 10 to 20 cc/kg/24 hr. Aspiration of volumes larger than this amount may require concurrent infusion of colloid.

10. Interruption of flow may indicate occlusion of the needle or catheter by tissue or debris. Manipulation of the catheter or repositioning the patient may help in locating another pocket of fluid. An alternate technique is to introduce a small volume of air to dislodge any occlusion.

11. Remove the needle or catheter and place a sterile gauze dressing.

COMPLICATIONS

1. Hemorrhage
2. Intravascular volume depletion with large volume paracentesis
3. Electrolyte abnormality (usually hyponatremia) with large-volume paracentesis, and negative nitrogen balance with repeated paracentesis
4. Perforation of bowel or other intra-abdominal organ
5. Peritonitis introduced by skin contamination or bowel perforation
6. Persistent leakage of peritoneal fluid, or dissection through fascial planes, resulting in scrotal or labial edema

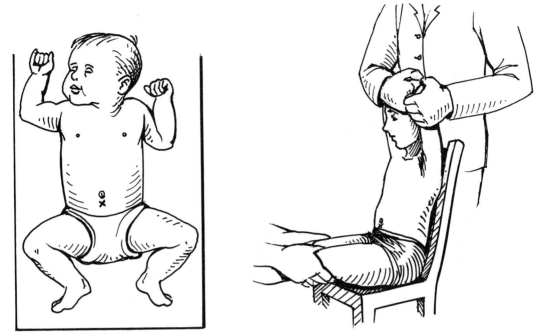

Figure 31-2. Paracentesis may also be performed in a supine frog-legged position or in older children may be performed upright. In these positions the preferred puncture site is in the midline below the umbilicus (indicated with an X).

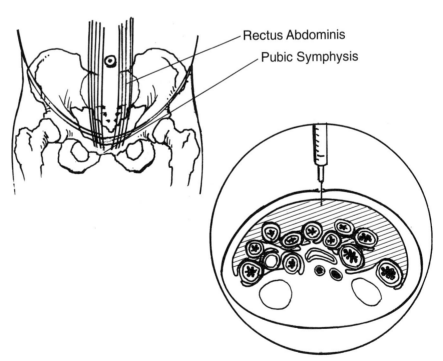

Rectus Abdominis

Pubic Symphysis

Figure 31-3. The abdominal wall is pierced with a needle or a catheter with a needle trochar. Maintain negative pressure on the syringe and halt the advance of the needle when a "pop" is felt.

References

Cabot EB. Abdominal paracentesis. In May HL, Aghababian RV, Fleisher GR (eds): *Emergency Medicine* (2nd ed). Boston, Little, Brown, 1992, pp 2180–2182.

Fitzgerald JF. Ascites. In Wyllie R, Hyams JS (eds): *Pediatric Gastrointestinal Disease.* Philadelphia, WB Saunders, 1993, pp 151–160.

Glauser JM. Paracentesis. In Roberts JR, Hedges JR (eds): *Clinical Procedures in Emergency Medicine* (2nd ed) Philadelphia, WB Saunders, 1991, pp 674–679.

Hoefs JC. Diagnostic paracentesis: A potent clinical tool. Gastroenterology 98:230–236, 1990.

Hoefs JC, Jonas GM. Diagnostic paracentesis. Adv Intern Med 37:391–409, 1992.

Hoffman DM, Martell AT. A new technique for therapeutic paracentesis. Surg Gynecol Obstetr 177:87–88, 1993.

Neighbor ML. Ascites. Emerg Med Clin North Am 7:683–697, 1989.

APPENDIX

INTERPRETATION OF PERITONEAL FLUID FINDINGS

Appearance: Normal fluid should have a clear, straw colored appearance. Cloudy fluid is present with infectious or inflammatory processes. Milky fluid is present with chylous ascites. Bloody fluid in the absence of trauma is consistent with malignant, tuberculous, or pancreatic ascites.

Cell count: A peritoneal fluid neutrophil count of $>250/\mu l$ in patients with signs of peritonitis and $>500/\mu l$ in any patient is consistent with bacterial infection. A mononuclear leukocytosis is present with tuberculous peritonitis.

Culture and Gram stain: These tests should be performed on all peritoneal fluid aspirates, although both may be negative in over 50% of cases. Interpretation is complicated by the occurrence of two entities, which may be identical to spontaneous bacterial peritonitis—bacterascites and culture-negative neutrocytic ascites. The former, by analogy to bacteriuria, represents peritoneal fluid colonization without leukocytosis. The latter represents failure to recover an organism in the presence of a peritoneal fluid leukocytosis. Yield may be improved by the immediate inoculation of blood culture bottles with 5 to 10 ml and the use of large-volume spun samples for Gram stain; concurrent blood cultures may be useful in this situation. The presence of mixed bacterial infection implies peritonitis secondary to bowel perforation.

Biochemical analysis:

Amylase: Elevated above serum levels in pancreatic ascites

Glucose: Depressed in tuberculous peritonitis (<30 mg/dl) and secondary peritonitis (<50 mg/dl)

Protein: Elevated (>2.5 to 3 g/dl) in so-called exudative processes such as infection and malignancy. Lower values are consistent with "transudative" ascites caused by cirrhosis, hemodynamic, or cardiovascular abnormalities, or nephrosis.

Lactate dehydrogenase (LDH): Elevated in exudative ascites. A peritoneal fluid-to-serum LDH ratio >0.5 also suggests an "exudative" fluid.

Albumin: The reliability of protein and LDH determinations in classifying the etiology of ascites has been questioned. The serum-to-ascites albumin concentration gradient is thought to be a more useful test in the differential diagnosis of ascites. Gradients >1.1 g/dl occur when portal venous pressures are elevated, as in cirrhosis or cardiac failure. Values <1.1 g/dl are consistent with "exudative" processes or decreases in oncotic pressure.

Lipids: Triglyceride level is elevated (>400 mg/dl) in chylous ascites.

Other: Cytologic and mycobacterial studies are performed as appropriate.

CHAPTER 32

Jim R. Harley

DIAGNOSTIC PERITONEAL LAVAGE

INDICATIONS

1. Unexplained shock, altered sensorium, or falling hematocrit in a blunt trauma patient
2. Major thoracic, neurosurgical, or orthopedic injury (fractured femur or pelvis) requiring emergent surgery

CONTRAINDICATIONS

1. Obvious need for emergency celiotomy
2. Previous abdominal surgeries (relative)

EQUIPMENT

1. Povidone-iodine solution
2. 1% lidocaine with epinephrine
3. Sterile towels
4. Sterile gloves
5. #15 scalpel blade
6. Curved hemostats
7. Retractors
8. Gauze
9. Ringer's lactated solution
10. Guidewire
11. Peritoneal catheter
12. Sutures
13. Introducer needle
14. 20- or 30-cc syringe

PROCEDURE (GUIDED WIRE TECHNIQUE)

1. Place the patient in a flat, supine position.
2. Decompress the bladder with a urethral catheter.
3. Decompress the stomach with a nasogastric tube.

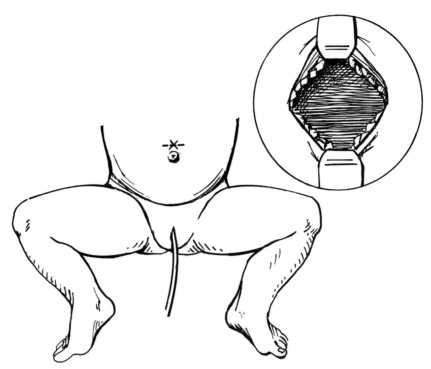

Figure 32–1. A diagnostic peritoneal lavage in a young child is performed superior to the umbilicus. A 1- to 2-cm incision is made down to the linea alba.

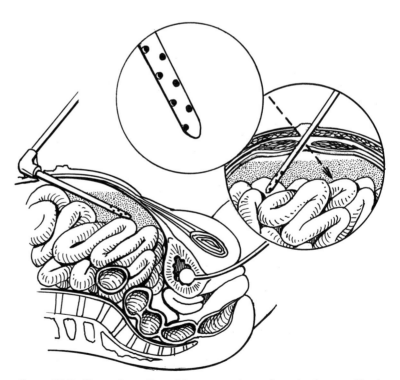

Figure 32–2. Diagnostic peritoneal lavage can be performed using a guidewire introducer technique. An introducer needle is inserted, the wire is threaded through. The needle is withdrawn and the peritoneal catheter (shown in place here) is passed over the guidewire, and the wire is withdrawn.

4. The insertion site is then prepped with Betadine and infiltrated with 1% lidocaine.
   a. Supraumbilical approach: This is recommended in small children. The insertion site is 1 to 2 cm above the umbilicus in the midline (Fig. 32-1).
   b. Infraumbilical approach: The site is recommended for larger children and adults. The insertion site is one third of the distance from the umbilicus to the symphysis pubis in the midline.
5. A 1.5- to 2-cm transverse incision is then made. The subcutaneous tissue is incised down to the linea alba (Fig. 32-1).
6. The introducer needle is then inserted through the linea alba and peritoneum and then directed inferiorly.
7. The guidewire is then inserted through the needle. The guidewire should advance easily toward the pelvis.
8. The introducer needle is then removed. Do not let go of the guidewire until it is removed from the patient.
9. The peritoneal catheter is then placed over the guidewire (Fig. 32-2).
10. The guidewire is then removed.
11. A syringe is then attached to the catheter and aspirated. If free blood is aspirated, this is considered a very positive result.
12. If free blood is not aspirated, infuse 10–20 ml/kg of Ringer's lactated solution though the catheter. Turn the patient from side to side to increase mixing. (C-spine precautions should be followed if there is a C-spine injury.)
13. The intravenous (IV) infusion bag is then placed below the patient to allow the infused fluid to flow out of the patient.
14. The recovered fluid should be sent for red and white blood cell counts.
15. The catheter is then removed and the incision closed with sutures.
16. A red blood cell (RBC) count of >100,000 per mm^3 is considered a positive result. A RBC count <50,000 per mm^3 is considered negative. A RBC count between 50,000 and 100,000 per mm^3 is considered equivocal.

PERCUTANEOUS THRUST TECHNIQUE

1. The skin is incised 2 to 3 cm in the same site as described for the guidewire technique with a #11 scalpel (Fig. 32-1).
2. A #9 Fr peritoneal lavage catheter with trocar inserted is placed through the incision (Fig. 32-3).
3. Once the catheter has passed through the peritoneum 0.5 to 1.0 cm, the trocar is pulled back and the catheter is directed into the right or left lower quadrant. (see Fig. 32-2).
4. Remove trochar. Follow steps 11 to 16 shown earlier.

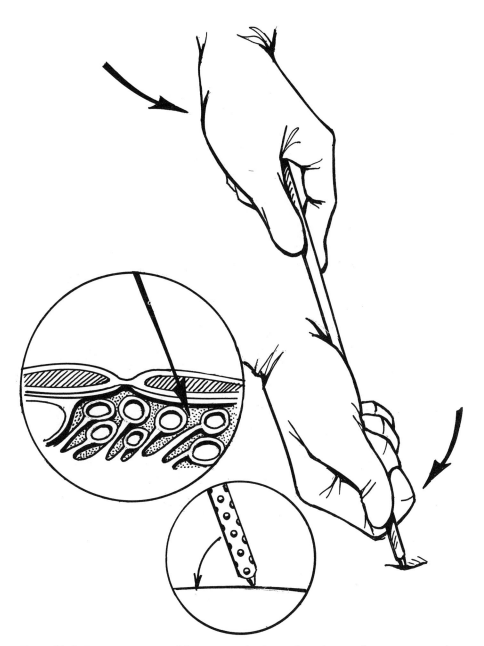

Figure 32–3. Diagnostic peritoneal lavage can also be performed using the percutaneous thrust technique. A peritoneal catheter with trochar is inserted through the incision. The left hand provides the pressure, while the right hand resists the pressure and limits the depth of insertion of the catheter.

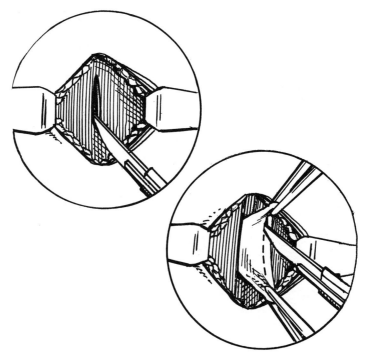

Figure 32–4. Diagnostic peritoneal lavage can also be performed using the mini-lap technique. A 3-cm long vertical incision is made, and the tissue bluntly dissected down to the linea alba which is then incised. The peritoneum is grasped in two hemostats and pulled into the wound. The peritoneum is incised and the catheter is inserted into this opening.

MINI-LAP TECHNIQUE

1. A vertical incision 3 to 5 cm long is made in the same location described in the guidewire technique (Fig. 32-4).
2. The tissue is bluntly dissected down to the linea alba. The linea alba is then incised (Fig. 32-4).
3. The peritoneum is then grasped with two hemostats through the opening in the linea alba. The peritoneal is then incised with a scalpel (Fig. 32-4).
4. The peritoneal catheter is then inserted.
5. Follow steps 12 to 16 shown earlier.
6. Once the lavage is done, the catheter is removed. The peritoneum, fascia, and subcutaneous tissue should be closed in a layered manner with 2-0 or 3-0 absorbable sutures. The skin is then closed with nonabsorbable sutures.

COMPLICATIONS

1. False-positive test result owing to bleeding caused by the procedure
2. Hemorrhage
3. Peritonitis
4. Bladder perforation
5. Bowel perforation
6. Mesentery vessel perforation
7. Aorta perforation
8. Wound infection

References

Coleridge ST, Bell C. Diagnostic peritoneal lavage. In Roberts JR, Hedges JR, (eds). *Clinical Procedures in Emergency Medicine* (2nd ed). Philadelphia, WB Saunders, 1991, pp 679-689.

CHAPTER 33

David E. Bank

CULDOCENTESIS

INDICATIONS

1. To confirm the diagnosis of ectopic pregnancy
2. To confirm the diagnosis of a ruptured viscus (corpus luteal cyst, appendix)
3. To assist in diagnosing intra-abdominal injuries to the liver or spleen or both
4. To aid in fluid collection in adolescents with a diagnosis of pelvic inflammatory disease

CONTRAINDICATIONS

1. Pelvic mass detectable on bimanual examination (tubo-ovarian abscess, appendiceal abscess, ovarian mass, and pelvic kidneys)
2. Retroverted uterus
3. Coagulopathy
4. Prepubertal females

EQUIPMENT

1. Betadine solution
2. Sterile water
3. Cottonballs
4. 4×4 gauze sponges
5. 1% lidocaine with epinephrine
6. Syringes (20 ml)
7. Ring sponge forceps
8. 25-gauge needle
9. 18-gauge spinal needle
10. Uterine cervical tenaculum
11. Bivalve vaginal speculum
12. Adjustable examination table, preferably with stirrups

PROCEDURE

Before beginning the culdocentesis procedure, the examiner should be familiar with the anatomy of the pelvic area. The rectouterine pouch (pouch of Douglas) is the most dependent intraperitoneal area in both the upright and supine positions. It is formed by reflections of the peritoneum as the peritoneum courses the posterior wall of the uterus and folds itself upward along the anterior wall of the rectum. The pouch of Douglas separates the upper portion of the rectum from the uterus and upper vagina. This pouch may normally contain a small amount of peritoneal fluid and loops of small intestine.

1. Adequate conscious sedation should be achieved when possible.
2. Once conscious sedation is achieved, the patient is placed in the lithotomy position. Reverse Trendelenburg positioning is also maintained in order to enhance intraperitoneal fluid collection into the pouch of Douglas.
3. A bimanual pelvic examination is performed before the procedure to identify the presence of a fixed pelvic mass and to assess the position of the uterus.
4. The bivalve vaginal speculum is inserted to provide proper visualization of the posterior vaginal wall and cervical os.
5. The uterine cervical tenaculum is used to grasp the posterior lip of the cervix below the cervical os in order to provide cervical elevation (Fig. 33-1). The elevation of the posterior lip of the cervix provides appropriate exposure of the puncture site and stabilizes the posterior wall of the vagina during subsequent needle puncture. This maneuver may also elevate a retroverted uterus from the pouch of Douglas.
6. Once adequate exposure of the posterior vaginal wall has been obtained with tension obtained between the cervical tenaculum and the inferior blade of the bivalve speculum, the vaginal wall in the area of the pouch of Douglas should be swabbed with Betadine.
7. Local anesthesia may be obtained using 1% lidocaine with epinephrine through

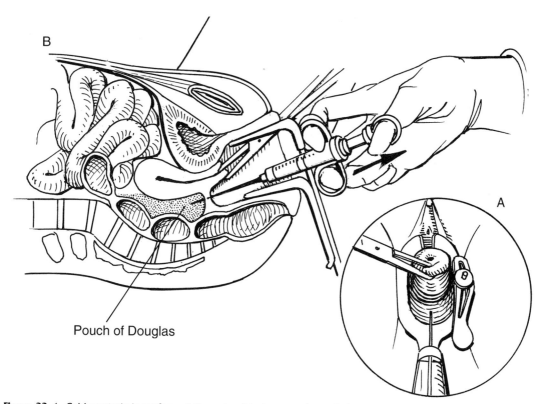

Pouch of Douglas

Figure 33–1. Culdocentesis is performed through a bivalve speculum. *A,* A uterine tenaculum is used to elevate the posterior lip of the cervix. *B,* Under local anesthesia, a spinal needle attached to a 20-cc syringe is inserted at 1 cm posterior to the point where the vaginal wall meets the cervix. The needle is inserted 2 to 2.5 cm into the pouch of Douglas, where fluid may be aspirated.

Table 33–1. **CULDOCENTESIS FLUID ANALYSIS**

Fluid	Interpretation
None or ≤0.3 ml of blood	Nondiagnostic
≤2 ml of clotted blood	Nondiagnostic
Clear (≤2 ml)	Normal
Clear, yellowish (≥2 ml, many WBCs)	Consider: Pelvic inflammatory disease
Purulent	Consider: Ruptured tubo-ovarian abscess Pelvic inflammatory disease Ruptured appendix
Bright red blood (or ≥0.3 ml of nonclotted blood)	Consider: Ruptured viscus or vascular injury Bleeding ectopic pregnancy (ruptured or unruptured)* Bleeding corpus luteum Intra-abdominal injury (liver, spleen, other)
Brown, nonclotted blood >2 ml	Consider: Chronic intraperitoneal bleeding from an ectopic pregnancy or organ/viscus injury

*The hematocrit of blood from a ruptured ectopic pregnancy is usually >15%.

a separate 25-gauge needle attached to a 20-cc syringe. The length of the 20-cc syringe allows the examiner to visualize the area of the vaginal wall to be punctured while also maintaining control of the needle.

8. After the local anesthetic is allowed to take effect, an 18-gauge, 1.5-in spinal needle attached to a 20-cc syringe filled with 2 to 3 ml of normal saline is advanced along the inferior blade of the speculum. Vaginal penetration should occur 1 to 1.5 cm posterior (inferior) to the point at which the vaginal wall meets the cervix (Fig. 33–1A, B).

9. Needle puncture should be performed at approximately 0 to 5 degrees to the coronal plane directed posteriorly. The needle should penetrate the inferior vaginal wall approximately 2 to 2.5 cm. The 2 to 3 ml of saline contained in the attached 20-cc syringe is expelled into the pouch of Douglas. The free flow of fluid from the syringe into the pouch of Douglas confirms that needle placement has not terminated in tissue such as the uterine wall or intestinal mucosa.

10. Negative pressure is applied to the syringe as the needle is slowly withdrawn from the retrouterine pouch. Care must be taken to avoid the aspiration of any blood that has accumulated in the vagina from cervical bleeding or previous needle insertions.

11. If no fluid is aspirated, the needle should be reintroduced and directed slightly to the right or left of the midline. The redirection of the needle should be 5 degrees or less to the sagittal plane, as a needle inserted too far laterally may result in a puncture of mesenteric or pelvic vessels.

12. Interpretation of results (Table 33–1).

COMPLICATIONS

1. Rupture of an unsuspected tubo-ovarian abscess
2. Perforation of bowel loops
3. Perforation of a pelvic kidney
4. Excessive bleeding in patients with a coagulopathy

References

Cunningham GF. *Williams Obstetrics* (19th ed). Norwalk, CT, Appleton & Lange, 1993, p 703.

Roberts JR, Hedges JR. *Clinical Procedures in Emergency Medicine*. Philadelphia, WB Saunders, 1991, pp 936–941.

Simon RR, Brenner BE. *Emergency Procedures and Techniques* (2nd ed). Baltimore, Williams & Wilkins, 1987, pp 189–190.

CHAPTER 34

David E. Bank and John T. Kanegaye

ARTHROCENTESIS

INDICATIONS

1. Synovial fluid analysis
2. Relief of severely symptomatic effusion
3. Therapeutic injection
4. Saline arthrogram for diagnosis of intra-articular involvement of adjacent laceration prior to repair

CONTRAINDICATIONS

1. Infection (cellulitis or abscess) overlying proposed puncture site
2. Bleeding diathesis or anticoagulant therapy (relative, as significant symptom relief may be obtained by drainage of hemarthrosis after correction of coagulopathy)
3. Adjacent fracture (relative, as the presence of fat globules in joint aspirate may establish the diagnosis of previously unsuspected intra-articular fracture)

EQUIPMENT

1. Supplies for asepsis
   a. Sterile drapes
   b. Sterile gloves
   c. Bactericidal solution (generally povidone-iodine) and alcohol swabs
   d. Shave kit for the hirsute patient
2. Anesthetic: Topical coolant (ethyl chloride), *or* 1% lidocaine for infiltration
3. Sterile syringes
   a. 1–3 ml for infiltration of anesthetic
   b. 10–20 ml for aspiration
4. Sterile needles
   a. 25-gauge for local anesthetic infiltration
   b. 18–20-gauge for aspiration, *or* over-the-needle catheter
5. Stopcock and/or short intravenous (IV) connecting tubing (optional adjuncts permitting changes of syringes and giving leeway for motion in the uncooperative patient)
6. Specimen collection tubes
   a. EDTA anticoagulant (lavender top, complete blood count [CBC] tube) for cell count
   b. Plain (red top) for chemistry, serology

c. Heparin (green top, preferably with liquid anticoagulant) for crystal analysis
d. Culture tubes for microbiologic studies
7. Sterile gauze sponges and dressing supplies

GENERAL APPROACH

1. For most joints, successful aspiration is more likely with:
   a. an approach along the extensor surface, where the joint capsule is more accessible and where intervening structures are less likely to be encountered
   b. slight flexion of the joint (except as detailed below) to widen the joint space
   c. axial traction along the joint
   d. compression around large joints to maximize accumulation of synovial fluid under the chosen puncture site
2. Strict attention to sterile technique is required. Paint the region around the proposed puncture site widely with povidone-iodine solution three times and allow it to dry. The dried scrub solution at the puncture site may be removed with an alcohol swab to prevent inadvertent introduction into the joint space or interference with microbiologic studies. Apply sterile drapes, and consider changing gloves after skin preparation.
3. Identify puncture site and deliver topical or infiltrated anesthesia.
4. Puncture the skin with a needle-syringe assembly and advance into the joint space, aspirating for fluid return. Several additional considerations are relevant at this stage:
   a. Although needle choice is limited by the size of the joint, the use of the largest possible needle will prevent occlusion by debris contained in the aspirated fluid.
   b. The use of an over-the-needle catheter is recommended by some authors to minimize the likelihood of trauma incurred by inadvertent needle movement.
   c. For evacuation of large effusions, the use of a large syringe or a stopcock (to facilitate changes of syringes) is recommended.
   d. The use of a short segment of IV tubing (T connector) between the needle and syringe may facilitate entry into the joint space and changes of syringes and will decrease the likelihood of inadvertent trauma to the joint when patient movement is anticipated. An alternative to this arrangement, especially for small joints, is a scalp vein needle.
5. Remove the maximum volume possible and save for analysis, if indicated. Two simple tests may be performed at bedside before formal laboratory analysis:
   a. The "string" sign, the bedside correlate of the mucin clot test, is elicited by expressing a drop of synovial fluid from its syringe. Fluid of normal viscosity should result in a string 5 to 10 cm long. Alternatively, a drop of fluid may be stretched between two gloved fingers. Reduction in viscosity reflects intra-articular inflammation.
   b. The presence of fat globules, visible when the aspirate is allowed to sit briefly on a nonporous surface, is suggestive of a fracture with intra-articular extension.
6. In the event of difficulty with aspiration of fluid, the following may be attempted:
   a. Careful manipulation of the needle or joint position, with caution to avoid laceration of the synovial membrane or scoring of the articular cartilage.
   b. Reduction of the amount of suction being applied to the syringe
   c. Use of a smaller syringe
   d. Reinjection of a small amount of previously aspirated fluid

e. Injection of a small volume of preservative-free saline solution, followed by aspiration of a mixture of saline and synovial fluid for analysis

f. Compression over other palpable aspects of the joint (e.g., compression over the suprapatellar pouch to "milk" additional fluid toward the needle)

7. Remove the needle and place a sterile gauze dressing over the puncture site.

COMPLICATIONS

1. Introduction of infection (from skin surface or during bacteremic episode)
2. Hemarthrosis
3. Laceration of synovium, cartilage, or adjacent structure (nerve, vessel, tendon)

SPECIFIC ANATOMIC SITES

The Shoulder

Anterior Approach

Joint Position. The arm is adducted with the patient seated.

Anatomic Landmarks. The coracoid process and the proximal humerus are identified at the anterior aspect of the shoulder (Fig. 34-1A).

Approach to Puncture. A 20-gauge needle is inserted lateral to the coracoid process and medial to the proximal humeral head directed posteriorly toward the glenoid rim (Fig. 34-1B). Care should be taken to avoid the thoracoacromial artery as it traverses the length of the coracoacromial ligament.

Posterior Approach

Joint Position. With the patient seated, the arm is adducted and internally rotated in order to tighten the posterior joint capsule (Fig. 34-2).

Anatomic Landmarks. The angle of the acromion is palpated posteriorly at the junction of the spine of the scapula and the acromion process. A concavity or depression in this area can frequently be appreciated (Fig. 34-3A).

Approach to Puncture. With the shoulder slightly internally rotated, the needle is inserted horizontally one fingerbreadth below the angle of the acromion. It traverses the posterior fibers of the deltoid muscle passing between the head of the humerus and the lip of the glenoid fossa (Fig. 34-3B). The needle is directed in an anteromedial direction at a 15-degree angle with the coronal plane. The advantage of this approach is the paucity of tendons and ligaments in this anatomic area.

The Elbow

Joint Position. The elbow is flexed 90 degrees with the forearm pronated.

Anatomic Landmarks. The head of the radius and the lateral epicondyle of the humerus may be more easily identified with extension of the elbow. Supination and pronation facilitate identification of the radial head (Fig. 34-4A).

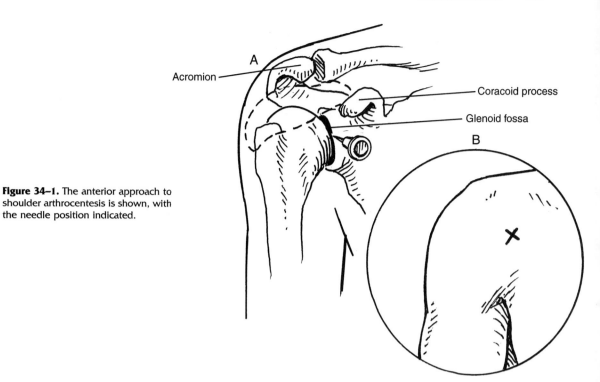

Acromion

Coracoid process

Glenoid fossa

Figure 34–1. The anterior approach to shoulder arthrocentesis is shown, with the needle position indicated.

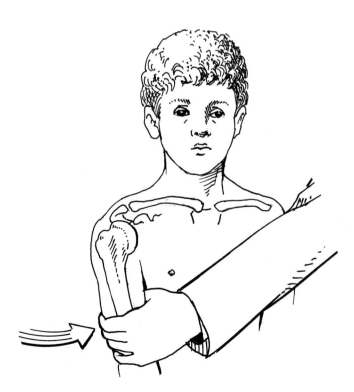

Figure 34–2. For the posterior approach to shoulder arthrocentesis to be performed, the patient must be seated with the arm adducted and internally rotated.

Approach to Puncture. A 22-gauge needle is inserted, directed medially, at the lateral aspect of the elbow in the groove formed by the lateral epicondyle and the radial head. Approaches medial to the olecranon are not recommended because of the presence of the superior ulnar collateral artery and, more importantly, the ulnar nerve. This approach can also be identified if one draws an imaginary triangle among the lateral epicondyle, the head of the radius, and the olecranon (Fig. 34-4B). Needle insertion is in the middle of the triangle, directed medially at a 90-degree angle to the humerus. The needle traverses the anconeus muscle into the joint space.

The Wrist

Joint Position. The wrist is flexed 20 to 30 degrees, with traction.

Anatomic Landmarks. The dorsal radial tubercle is palpated on the dorsal aspect of the distal radius. This landmark is located ulnar to both the extensor pollicis longus tendon and the "anatomic snuff box," which should be avoided as it contains the radial artery and superior radial nerve (Fig. 34-5).

Approach to Puncture. A 22-gauge needle is inserted at the dorsal aspect of the wrist in a palmar direction. Insertion is in an area enclosed by the dorsal radial tubercle, the carpal lunate bone, and the extensor tendons of the extensor digitorum communis muscle and the extensor pollicis longus muscle (Fig. 34-5).

The Interphalangeal and Metacarpophalangeal Joints

Joint Position. The joint is flexed approximately 15 to 20 degrees with traction.

Anatomic Landmarks. For the metacarpophalagneal (MP) joint, the space between the metacarpal head and the prominence at the proximal end of the proximal phalanx is identified. The proximal and distal interphalangeal (IP) joints lie just distal to the dorsal skin creases of the finger. The extensor tendon runs down the dorsal midline and should be avoided (Fig. 34-6).

Approach to Puncture. A 22-gauge needle is inserted into the joint space dorsally, in a palmar direction, either medial or lateral to the extensor tendon (Fig. 34-6).

The First Carpometacarpal (Radiocarpal) Joint

Joint Position. The thumb is apposed against the fifth finger to expose the proximal end of the first metacarpal. Traction may also be helpful.

Anatomic Landmarks. The radial aspect of the proximal first metacarpal may be found just palmar to the abductor pollicis longus (APL) tendon. Just dorsal and proximal to this tendon is the "anatomic snuffbox," which should be avoided (Fig. 34-7).

Approach to Puncture. A 22-gauge needle is inserted on the palmar side proximal to the base of the first metacarpal pointing in an ulnar direction (Fig. 34-7).

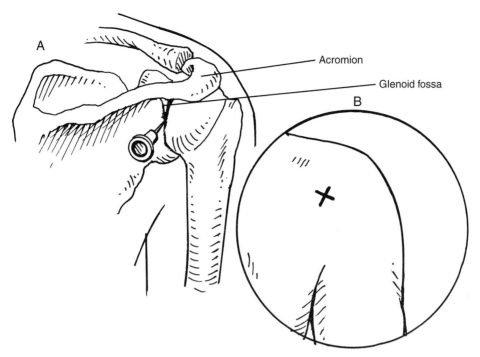

Figure 34–3. The posterior approach to shoulder arthrocentesis is shown with the needle position indicated.

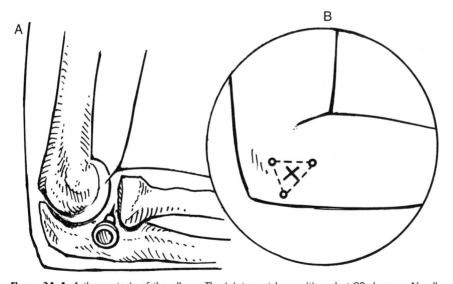

Figure 34–4. Arthrocentesis of the elbow. The joint must be positioned at 90 degrees. Needle insertion site is shown.

The Hip

Although techniques are described for aspiration of this joint, the authors feel that this procedure is best performed with fluoroscopic guidance (and optimally using deep sedation or a general anesthetic technique) and thus is not suitable outside the pediatric operating suite.

The Knee

Parapatellar Approach

Joint Position. The knee is fully extended with the patient supine.

Anatomic Landmarks. The posterior border of the patella (inferior with the patient supine) and the groove of the femorotibial articulation are palpable on both the medial and lateral aspects of the knee (Fig. 34-8).

Approach to Puncture. Holding the needle parallel to the table (or slightly above parallel, with the syringe elevated 10 to 20 degrees), puncture the skin on the medial or lateral aspect of the knee in the space below the inferior border of the patella and above the femorotibial articulation (Fig. 34-8).

Anatomic Consideration. Although proponents exist for medial and lateral approaches, a lateral approach avoids interference from the contralateral extremity as well as the possible need to penetrate the vastus medialis muscle. The suprapatellar bursa often communicates with the joint space and may be "milked" down to distend the joint. The superior and inferior genicular arteries form anastomoses in this region; however, vascular injury is not common and may be minimized by aspiration during needle puncture and advancement. For all approaches to the knee, one should be prepared for a potentially large-volume aspirate.

Infrapatellar Approach

Joint Position. The knee is in 90 degrees of flexion over the edge of the table.

Anatomic Landmarks. The patellar tendon, inferior to the inferior pole of the patella (Fig. 34-9).

Approach to Puncture. Approaching anteriorly to the flexed knee with the needle perpendicular to the tendon, puncture through the middle of the patellar tendon or just lateral to it, penetrating through the underlying fat and into the joint space between the femoral condyles (Fig. 34-9).

Anatomic Consideration. Although this approach is not the most commonly used, advantages include a widened joint surface for needle entry, decreased risk of scoring the articular cartilage, and relative paucity of pain fibers in the needle path. It is also useful when the knee cannot be brought into full extension.

Suprapatellar Approach

Joint Position. Knee in extension with patient supine

Anatomic Landmarks. Groove between the patella and lateral femoral condyle under the superolateral corner of the patella (Fig. 34-10).

Approach to Puncture. With the needle parallel to the table, puncture the skin just inferior and lateral to the superolateral corner of the patella. Advance into the joint space in a direction perpendicular to the leg or in a slightly inferomedial direction (Fig. 34-10).

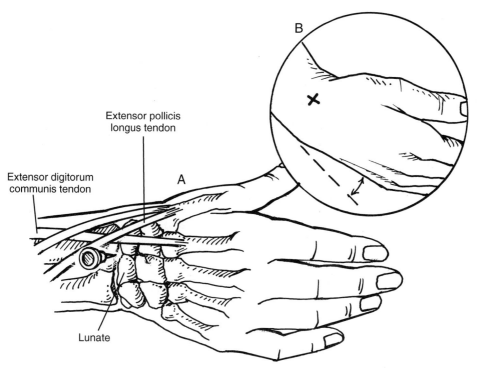

Extensor pollicis
longus tendon

Extensor digitorum
communis tendon

A

B

Lunate

Figure 34–5. Arthrocentesis of the wrist is facilitated by flexing the wrist 20 to 30 degrees. Needle insertion site is shown.

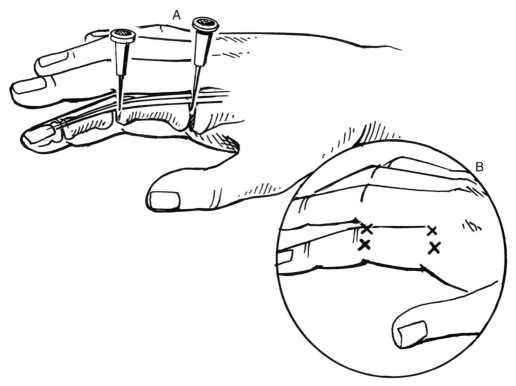

A

B

Figure 34–6. Needle insertion sites for interphalangeal and metacarpophalangeal joints are shown.

Anatomic Consideration. The suprapatellar bursa may contain little fluid or may not communicate with the joint space in some patients. The approach is ideal, however, if this bursa is well distended.

The Ankle

Anteromedial Approach

Joint Position. Foot in plantar flexion with patient supine

Anatomic Landmarks. The joint space of the tibiotalar articulation is palpated as a depression anterior and lateral to the medial malleolus. The puncture site is medial to the tendon of either the extensor hallucis longus (EHL) or the tibialis anterior (TA). These tendons are readily palpable with the foot in 90 degrees of dorsiflexion, with the EHL tendon demonstrated by active extension of the great toe and the TA tendon by active inversion of the foot. After identifying the landmark tendon, the foot is brought into plantar flexion to widen the joint space (Fig. 34-11).

Approach to Puncture. Directing the needle perpendicular to the examination table (in a downward vertical direction), puncture the skin medial to the tendon of the EHL or the TA (depending on where the larger space exists) into the space palpable distal to the edge of the tibia (Fig. 34-11).

Anatomic Precaution. The dorsalis pedis artery and the deep peroneal nerve run just lateral to the EHL tendon, and the saphenous vein runs along the anterior surface of the medial malleolus.

Anterolateral Approach

Joint Position. As described earlier

Anatomic Landmarks. The tibiotalar articulation is palpable as a sulcus anterior and medial to the distal end of the fibula. The medial border of this sulcus at this location is formed by the tendon the peroneus tertius muscle, which is made more prominent by active dorsiflexion and eversion of the foot.

Approach to Puncture. Puncture the skin over the tibiotalar articulation lateral to the peroneus tertius tendon and direct the needle toward the medial malleolus.

Anatomic Consideration. This approach is less optimal, as a smaller space is presented and the perforating branch of the peroneal artery and the lateral anterior malleolar artery run along the anterior surface of the lateral malleolus.

Metatarsophalangeal (MTP) Joint

Joint Position. Neutral position or slight flexion with axial traction

Anatomic Landmarks. The joint space between the metatarsal head and the base of the proximal phalanx is palpable along the dorsal surface on either side of the extensor tendon (Fig. 34-12).

Approach to Puncture. Holding the needle perpendicular to the skin of the toe, puncture the skin adjacent to the extensor tendon into the MTP joint space. For the great toe, greater space is found medial to the EHL tendon. For other MTP joints, puncture may be performed medial or lateral to the tendon of the extensor digitorum longus (Fig. 34-12).

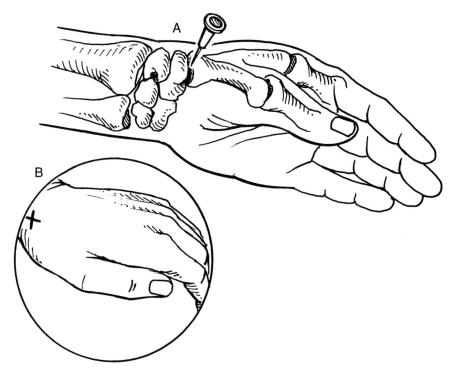

Figure 34–7. Arthrocentesis of the first carpometacarpal joint is facilitated by placing the thumb and little finger in apposition. Needle insertion sites are shown.

Figure 34–8. Arthrocentesis of the knee can be approached in three different ways. Illustrated here is the parapatellar approach. The knee is positioned in full extension, and the needle is inserted parallel to the table.

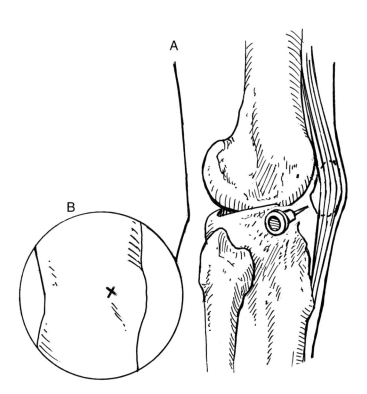

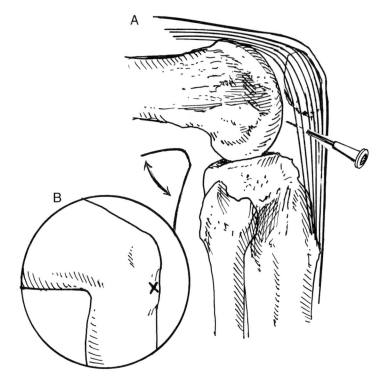

Figure 34–9. In the infrapatellar approach to arthrocentesis of the knee, the knee is positioned in 90 degrees of flexion and the needle is inserted in the middle of the patellar tendon. This approach is less commonly used.

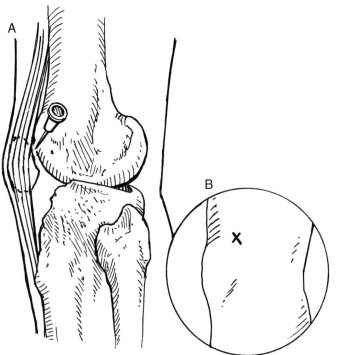

Figure 34–10. The suprapatellar approach to arthrocentesis of the knee is performed with the knee in full extension. It offers an ideal approach when the suprapatellar bursa is distended with fluid.

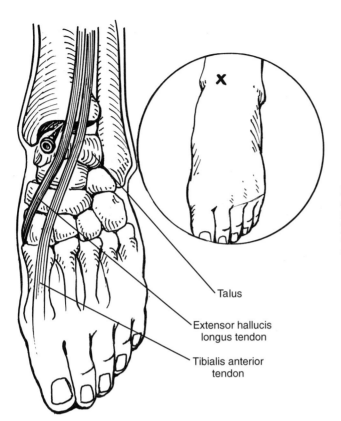

Figure 34–11. The anteromedial approach to ankle arthrocentesis is shown here. The joint is held in extension and eversion to maximize the joint space. The needle is inserted medial to either the extensor hallucis longus or the tibialis anterior.

Talus

Extensor hallucis longus tendon

Tibialis anterior tendon

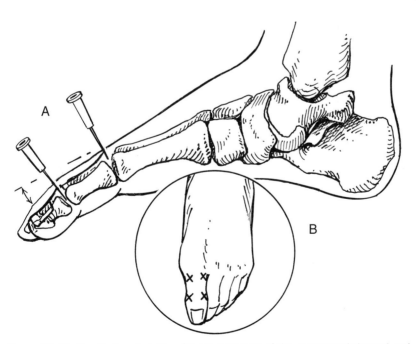

Figure 34–12. Needle insertion sites for arthrocentesis of the metatarsophalangeal and interphalangeal joints are shown.

Anatomic Consideration. The paired dorsal digital arteries and nerves run along the digit lateral to the puncture site.

Interphalangeal (IP) Joints

Joint Position. As for MTP aspiration
Anatomic Landmarks. The IP joint space lies in the bony prominence formed by the widening of the phalanges at their proximal and distal ends (Fig. 34-12).
Approach to Puncture. As for MTP aspiration (Fig. 34-12)
Anatomic Consideration. As for MTP aspiration

References

Ezell SL, Kobernick ME, Benjamin GC. Arthrocentesis. In Roberts JR, Hedges JR (eds.). *Clinical Procedures in Emergency Medicine* (2nd ed). Philadelphia, WB Saunders, 1991, pp 847-859.
Kasser JR. Bone and joint infections. In Canale ST, Beaty JH (eds). *Operative Pediatric Orthopedics*. St. Louis, Mosby-Year Book, 1991, pp 1047-1071.
Simon RR, Brenner BE. Orthopedic procedures. In *Emergency Procedures and Techniques* (2nd ed). Baltimore, Williams & Wilkins, 1987, pp 192-243.
Talbot-Stern JK. Arthritis, tendinitis, and bursitis. In Rosen P, Barkin RM, Braen GR, et al (eds). *Emergency Medicine: Concepts and Clinical Practice* (3rd ed). St. Louis, Mosby-Year Book, 1992, pp 804-828.
Warner WC. Infectious arthritis. In Crenshaw AH (ed). *Campbell's Operative Orthopaedics* (8th ed). St. Louis, Mosby-Year Book, 1992, pp 151-175.

APPENDIX

SYNOVIAL FLUID ANALYSIS

The accumulation of fluid in the joint space occurs secondary to inflammation of the synovial membrane, leading to the extravasation of an ultradialysate of plasma into the joint. Depending on the etiology of the effusion, the degree of inflammation may be classified as minimal, moderate, or severe. The use of appearance, leukocyte count with differential, Gram's stain, glucose and protein determinations, and the mucin clot test helps to determine the degree of inflammation and the most likely etiologies for the effusion (Table 34-1).

Appearance. Normal synovial fluid is straw-colored. With inflammatory changes, the fluid assumes a darker yellow to greenish hue. Grossly bloody fluid

Table 34–1. **SYNOVIAL FLUID ANALYSIS**

Disease	Appearance	WBC (#/μl)	PMN (%)	Glucose (% of serum)	Culture
None	Clear	<200	<25	95–100	Negative
Traumatic	Straw-colored, bloody, or xanthochromic	10–2000	<25	95–100	Negative
Rheumatoid, immune-mediated	Turbid	2000–50,000	50–75	≈75	Negative
Septic	Turbid, purulent	5000≥50,000	>75	<50	May be positive

suggests trauma, although defects in coagulation must be considered. Turbidity reflects cellularity as well as the presence of crystals and cartilaginous debris.

Bedside Tests. The fluid may be assessed for the "string sign" and the presence of fat globules immediately after being obtained (refer to "General Approach" for technique).

Cell Count. Normal leukocyte count is 10 to 200/μl, although up to 2000/μl may be seen in traumatic, noninflammatory effusions. In moderate inflammatory reactions, as seen in arthritides of immune-mediated origin, counts range from 2000 to 50,000/μl. With severe inflammatory reactions, as seen in septic arthritis, leukocyte counts of greater than 50,000/μl are usually seen. However, cell counts significantly lower than 50,000/μl have occurred with septic arthritis. In general, there are greater than 75% polymorphonuclear cells with septic effusions.

Biochemical. Normal glucose levels in synovial fluid are 10 mg/dl less than serum. Protein values are usually 1.8 g/dl less than serum. The mucin clot test is a test of the quality of hyaluronic acid in fluid. Glacial acetic acid is added to a small amount of synovial fluid, forming a clot as it interacts with intact hyaluronic acid. With inflammation, the resulting clot is easily broken up.

Microbiologic. A Gram's stain and culture of synovial fluid are mandatory to exclude infectious etiologies. However, because of the bacteriostatic qualities of synovial fluid, these studies may be negative in septic arthritis, and extra-articular studies (blood culture, antigen studies) may prove useful in identifying an etiologic agent. In the presence of a negative culture, the most reliable synovial fluid findings seen in septic arthritis are a leukocyte count greater than 50,000/μl, a glucose concentration less than 50% of serum, and an elevated protein concentration. These findings may be particularly helpful in a child who has previously received antibiotics, making Gram's stain and culture less reliable.

CHAPTER 35

Michele Walsh-Sukys

SUPRAPUBIC BLADDER ASPIRATION

INDICATIONS

1. Obtaining sterile urine for culture
2. Draining a distended bladder with uretheral obstruction

CONTRAINDICATIONS

1. Infection of the skin over the pubis symphysis
2. Documented void within the preceding 1 hr
3. Abdominal distention
4. Abdominal anomalies
5. Genitourinary anomalies
6. Bleeding disorders

EQUIPMENT

1. Sterile gloves
2. Sterile drapes
3. Betadine
4. 3-cc syringe
5. 25-gauge straight needle, 1.5 in long
6. Band-Aid

TECHNIQUE

1. Have an assistant restrain the infant's legs.
2. Document that the infant has not voided for more than 1 hr before the attempt. This can be done by checking for a dry diaper or by applying a urine collection bag to the infant for 1 hr before the procedure.
3. Prepare the area between the pubis symphysis and the umbilicus with Betadine, and allow to dry.
4. Attach the needle to the syringe.
5. Insert the needle 1 to 1.5 cm above the pubis symphysis (there is frequently a

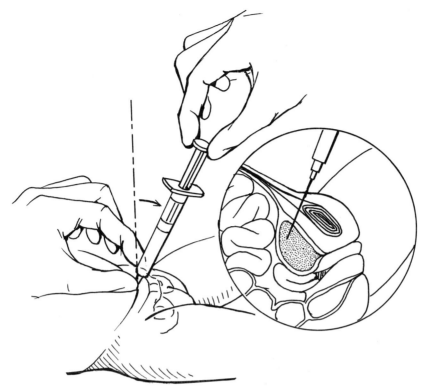

Figure 35-1. Insert the needle at the skinfold above the symphysis pubis with an angle that is 45 degrees from perpendicular, with the needle directed toward the head. While holding negative pressure on the syringe, advance the needle until urine is obtained.

skinfold in this area) 45 degrees below the perpendicular to the abdominal wall while withdrawing on the plunger (Fig. 35-1).

6. Insert the needle until urine is obtained, or approximately 1 cm in a preterm baby and 2 cm in a term baby.

7. If no urine is obtained on the first attempt, the procedure is terminated. There is no benefit, but considerable risk, to repeated attempts or blind probing.

8. Some authors have reported using ultrasound to enhance the chances of obtaining a successful tap, but ultrasound examination is rarely available in clinical use.

COMPLICATIONS

1. Hematuria: Microscopic hematuria is a frequent occurrence following suprapubic aspiration and is not clinically important. Less frequently gross hematuria may be seen and must be monitored closely.

2. Suprapubic hematoma is rarely seen.

3. Puncture of the bowel: If the bladder is not full, it is possible to enter the bowel. This may lead to contamination of the peritoneum, but the puncture usually seals spontaneously without difficulty.

Reference

Newman CG, O'Neill P, Parker A. Pyuria in infancy and the role of suprapubic bladder aspiration of urine in diagnosis of infection of the urinary tract. Br Med J 2:277, 1967.

CHAPTER 36

Brenda R. Hook

LUMBAR PUNCTURE

INDICATIONS

1. To confirm the diagnosis or cause of many diseases that may affect the brain, meninges, and spinal fluid, including suspected meningitis, neurosyphilis, seizures, encephalitis, or malignancy
2. To relieve increased intraventricular pressure and hydrocephalus caused by intraventricular hemorrhage, meningitis, malformations, or tumors. Lumbar punctures may need to be done serially in infants with progressive hydrocephalus.
3. Installation of intrathecal chemotherapy

CONTRAINDICATIONS

1. Defect or mass associated with the spine; neurosurgical consultation suggested
2. Should be delayed in patients who are in critical or unstable condition
3. Suspected elevated intracranial pressure in any pediatric patient. Herniation of the brainstem and cerebellum is extremely rare in the newborn period because of the presence of open sutures and fontanelles. If elevated intracranial pressure is suspected, a computed tomography (CT) scan should be performed before the tap.
4. Infection in skin overlying site
5. Bleeding diathesis (relative contraindication)

EQUIPMENT

1. Sterile and fenestrated drape
2. Sterile cap, mask, and gloves
3. Betadine solution
4. Sterile 2 × 2 gauze sponges
5. Four sterile collecting tubes
6. 1% lidocaine
7. 1-cc syringe with 25-gauge needle
8. Washcloth
9. Band-Aid
10. Spinal needle: 22 g. 1.5 in for infants; 21 g. 2.5 in for children; 20 g. 3.5 in for adolescents
11. Manometer

TECHNIQUE

1. The most important person in the success of this procedure is the assistant holding the patient. A few moments spent instructing the assistant before starting will save time, effort, and trauma for all involved.
2. Lumbar punctures may be done with the infant in the left or right lateral decubitus (left lateral decubitus is easier for a right-handed person) or the sitting position. In either situation the assistant will curl the patient into a fetal position. Make sure the spine is not twisted and forms a 90-degree angle with an imaginary line drawn through the hips. In the lateral decubitus position a perpendicular line should be present between an imaginary line drawn through both the hips and the table. Proper positioning is the most important aspect of technique in this procedure (Fig. 36–1). An older child may prefer to sit upright and lean on a bedside table.
3. Locate the ileal crests and draw a line through the spine. This line should cross the spine at the level of L4. Locate the first vertebral space caudal to this line.
4. Apply cap, mask, and gloves.
5. Apply Betadine to the lower back area. Allow to dry.

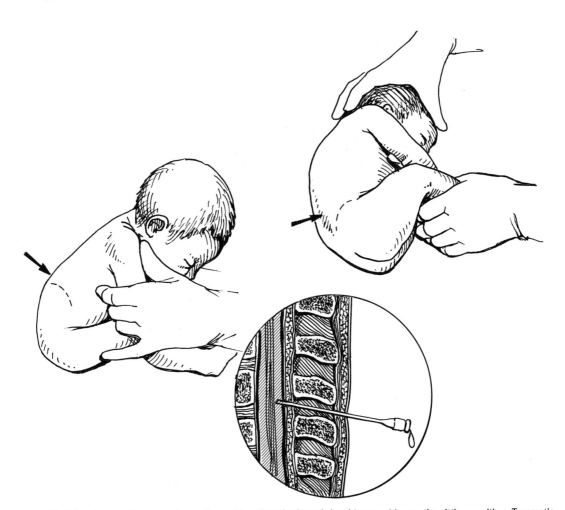

Figure 36–1. Lumbar puncture may be performed in either the lateral decubitus position or the sitting position. Traumatic lumbar punctures are most frequently caused by needle insertion that punctures the venous plexus posterior to the canal.

6. Create a sterile field by placing a drape on the table slightly under the infant's buttocks. Place the fenestrated drape so that the window is over the L4-L5 interspace.
7. Remove the Betadine from the immediate area using a sterile gauze sponge.
8. Check equipment to make sure spinal needle is functional and collecting tubes are open and easily available.
9. Place the thumb of your nondominant hand on the spinous process of L4.
10. Inject a small (0.1 to 0.2 ml) amount of 1% lidocaine over the L2-L3, L3-L4, or L4-L5 interspace.
11. Insert the needle, with the bevel up, into the skin over the desired interspace.
12. Slowly advance the entire needle while aiming for the umbilicus. Some resistance will be felt while going through the supraspinous and interspinous ligaments. A cessation of this pressure, and sometimes a small "pop," may be felt when the dura mater and arachnoid mater are pierced (Fig. 36-1).
13. Remove the stylet from the needle and observe for flow of cerebrospinal fluid (CSF). Rotation of the needle bevel toward the head may facilitate drainage.
14. With the aid of an assistant, attach a manometer to the needle and measure the opening pressure.
15. Collect 3 to 5 ml of spinal fluid into sterile tubes for culture analysis, glucose, protein, cell count and differential, antigen detection tests, and cytospin (if there is suspected malignancy).
16. One should *never* attempt to augment CSF flow by applying pressure to the open anterior fontanelle, or by aspirating fluid from the needle with a syringe. Such attempts may create a subdural hematoma.

COMPLICATIONS

1. Sudden decompression of elevated intracranial pressure resulting in herniation of cerebral tissue through tentorium or foramen magnum
2. Cardiopulmonary arrest related to either herniation or to hypoxemia induced by the knee-chest position
3. Infection
   a. Spinal or epidural abscesses
   b. Vertebral osteomyelitis
   c. Induced meningitis by lumbar puncture performed during bacteremia
4. Hemorrhage, subdural or subarachnoid
   a. Spinal epidural hematoma
   b. Intracranial, subdural, or subarachnoid hematoma
   c. Contamination of CSF sample by blood from puncture of the venous plexus or the posterior epidural surface
5. Intraspinal epidermoid tumor created when epithelial tissue is introduced into spinal canal. This complication can be avoided or reduced by using a spinal needle containing a trochar that prevents introduction of a "core biopsy" of tissue.
6. Neurologic injury
   a. Spinal cord puncture with nerve root injury if puncture site is above L2
   b. Paresthesia secondary to nerve root injury

References

Batnitzky S, Keucher TR, Mealey J, Campbell RL. Iatrogenic intraspinal epidermoid tumors. JAMA 237:148-150, 1977.

Bergman I, Wald ER, Meyer JD, Painter MJ. Epidural abscess and vertebral osteomyelitis following serial lumbar punctures. Pediatrics 72:476–478, 1983.

Blade J, Gaston F, Montserrat E, et al. Spinal subarachnoid hematoma after lumbar puncture causing reversible paraplegia in acute leukemia. J Neurosurg 58:438–440, 1983.

Dykes FD, Dunbar B, Lazarra A, Ahmann PA. Posthemorrhagic hydrocephalus in high-risk preterm infants: Natural history, management, and long-term outcome. J Pediatr 114:611–614, 1989.

Eldadah M, Frenkel LD, Hiatt IM, Heyi T. Evaluation of routine lumbar punctures in newborn infants with respiratory distress syndrome. Pediatr Infect Dis J 6:243–246, 1987.

Eng RHK, Seligman SJ. Lumbar puncture-induced meningitis. JAMA 245:1456–1460, 1981.

Fielkow S, Reuter S, Gotoff SP. Cerebrospinal fluid examination in symptom-free infants with risk factors for infection. J Pediatr 119:971–973, 1991.

Gleason CA, Martin RJ, Anderson JV, et al. Optimal position for a spinal tap in preterm infants. Pediatrics 71:31–36, 1983.

Hart IK, Bone I, Hadley DM. Development of neurological problems after lumbar puncture. Br Med J 296:51–53, 1988.

Hendricks-Muñoz KD, Shapiro DL. The role of the lumbar puncture in the admission sepsis evaluation of the premature infant. J Perinatol 10:60–64, 1990.

Kreusser KL, Tarby TJ, Kovnar E, et al. Serial lumbar punctures for at least temporary amelioration of neonatal posthemorrhagic hydrocephalus. Pediatrics 75:719–724, 1985.

Papile L-A, Burstein J, Burstein R, et al. Posthemorrhagic hydrocephalus in low-birth weight infants: Treatment by serial lumbar punctures. J Pediatr 97:273–277, 1980.

Porter FL, Miller JP, Cole FS, Marshall RE. A controlled clinical trial of local anesthesia for lumbar punctures in newborns. Pediatrics 88:663, 1991.

Rifaat M, El-Shafei I, Samra K, Sorour O. Intramedullary spinal abscess following spinal puncture. J Neurosurg 38:366–368, 1973.

Schwesenski J, McIntyre L, Bauer CR. Lumbar puncture frequency and cerebrospinal fluid analysis in the neonate. Am J Dis Child 145:54–58, 1991.

Shaywitz BA. Epidermoid spinal cord tumors and previous lumbar punctures. J Pediatr 80:638–640, 1972.

Smith KM, Deddish RB, Ogata ES. Meningitis associated with serial lumbar punctures and posthemorrhagic hydrocephalus. J Pediatr 109:1057–1060, 1986.

Spahr RC, MacDonald HM, Mueller-Heubach E. Knee-chest position and neonatal oxygenation and blood pressure. Am J Dis Child 135:79–81, 1981.

Teele DW, Dashefsky B, Rakusan T, Klein JO. Meningitis after lumbar puncture in children with bacteremia. N Engl J Med 305:1079–1083, 1981.

Ventriculomegaly Trial Group. Randomized trial of early tapping in neonatal posthemorrhagic ventricular dilatation. Arch Dis Child 65:3–6, 1990.

Weisman LE, Merenstein GB, Steenbarger JR. The effect of lumbar puncture position in sick neonates. Am J Dis Child 137:1077–1080, 1983.

Weiss MG, Ionides SP, Anderson CL. Meningitis in premature infants with respiratory distress: Role of admission lumbar puncture. J Pediatr 119:973–975, 1991.

CHAPTER 37

David E. Bank

TYMPANOCENTESIS

INDICATIONS

1. Immunocompromised children with acute otitis media with effusion
2. Acute otitis media with effusion resistant to multiple courses of antibiotic treatment
3. Immediate relief of severe pain caused by otitis media
4. Otitis media with effusion in the neonate
5. Otitis media with effusion complicated by suppurative processes (mastoiditis, meningitis, or brain abscess)

CONTRAINDICATIONS

1. Bleeding diathesis

EQUIPMENT

1. Papoose restraint
2. Dacron swab or ear curette
3. Otoscope with operating head
4. 1-cc tuberculin syringe
5. 22-gauge, 10-cm spinal needle
6. Sterile field
7. Mask, gown, and sterile gloves
8. Sterile gauze
9. Normal saline
10. Betadine solution

PROCEDURE

1. The indications and risks of the procedure should be explained to both the child and family.

Figure 37–1. Tympanocentesis is performed under direct visualization through an operating otoscope. The needle insertion sites are in the posterior or inferior quadrants of the tympanic membrane.

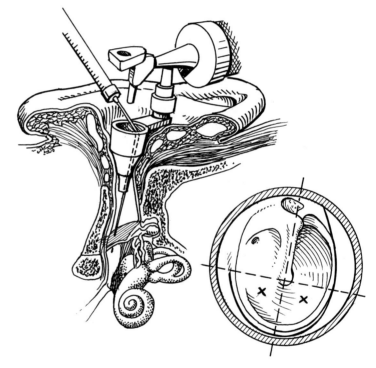

2. Adequate conscious sedation should be achieved whenever possible.
3. Once conscious sedation has been achieved, the child should be carefully placed in a papoose restraint in the supine position with the head held in the horizontal plane by an assistant.
4. With an otoscope with an operating head or an operating microscope, cerumen and debris should be evacuated, using direct visualization. Gentle use of a well-lubricated Dacron swab may assist in adequate visualization of the tympanic membrane.
5. The ear canal is sterilized by using a 9:1 diluted Betadine solution, administered for 1 to 2 min and then drained by turning the patient's head 180 degrees.
6. Once a sterile field has been created, the tympanic membrane should be revisualized using a handheld otoscope with operating head or an operating microscope. Puncture should be performed either with an 8- to 10-cm long, 22-gauge spinal needle bent 30 degrees, 4 to 5 cm from the distal end, or with a prepackaged tympanocentesis needle. A 1-ml tuberculin syringe should be attached to the needle (Fig. 37-1).
7. The needle is inserted via direct visualization in the posteroinferior quadrant of the membrane. This area corresponds to a region 1 to 2 mm from the distal portion of the handle of the malleus bone (Fig. 37-1).
8. As the middle ear is entered, aspiration should be performed with the tuberculin syringe. If less than 0.5 ml of fluid is obtained, consider flushing the needle with nonbacteriostatic normal saline solution.
9. After fluid is obtained, an assistant may help disengage the original tuberculin syringe so it may be sent to the laboratory with a sterile cap for Gram's stain and culture. The same assistant may then reattach a second tuberculin syringe to aid in needle withdrawal. Should no assistant be available, care must be taken in removing the original needle/tuberculin syringe apparatus, because contaminants from either the external ear canal or the otoscopic speculum may interfere with culture analysis.
10. Once aspiration is complete, the patient's tympanic membrane should again be visualized for any signs of excessive bleeding.

COMPLICATIONS

1. Bleeding
2. Evulsion of the tympanic membrane
3. Laceration of the external auditory canal
4. Disarticulation of the ossicular chain
5. Contamination of middle ear by infectious agents from the otoscopic speculum or external auditory canal

References

Bluestone CD, Stool SE. *Atlas of Pediatric Otolaryngology.* Philadelphia, WB Saunders, 1995, pp 29-30.
Fleisher GR, Ludwig S (eds). *Textbook of Pediatric Emergency Medicine* (3rd ed). Baltimore, Williams & Wilkins, 1993, pp 1601-1602.

CHAPTER 38

Timothy Mapstone and Patty Batchelder

ASSESSMENT OF VENTRICULAR SHUNT FUNCTION

INDICATIONS

1. For assessment of shunt function
2. To rule out elevated intracranial pressure

CONTRAINDICATIONS

None

EQUIPMENT

None (see Chapter 39, Ventricular Shunt Puncture)

PROCEDURE

1. Before the evaluation of shunt function is done, a general review of ventricular anatomy (Fig. 38-1), shunt anatomy, and mechanics may be beneficial.
   a. Ventricular catheter
      1. The tip is generally located in the body of the ventricle or the frontal horn (Fig. 38-2).
      2. Skull location is generally
         A. Just anterior and lateral to coronal suture
         B. Approximately 2.5 cm above and 2.5 cm behind top of ear
         C. Approximately 3 cm above and 2 cm lateral to the inion
      3. Most have a dome-shaped tapping reservoir, sometimes referred to as a Richham or Ommaya reservoir (there are many brand names), attached directly to the catheter and seated in a bur hole in the skull (Figs. 38-2, 38-3).
      4. Some tapping reservoirs are connected by a tube to the ventricular catheters, do not lie over the bur hole, and may be a part of the valve mechanism.

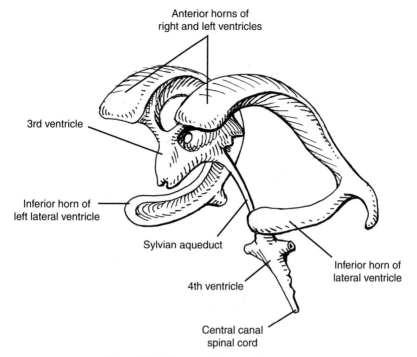

Anterior horns of
right and left ventricles

3rd ventricle

Inferior horn of
left lateral ventricle

Sylvian aqueduct

4th ventricle

Inferior horn of
lateral ventricle

Central canal
spinal cord

Figure 38–1. Diagram of ventricular anatomy.

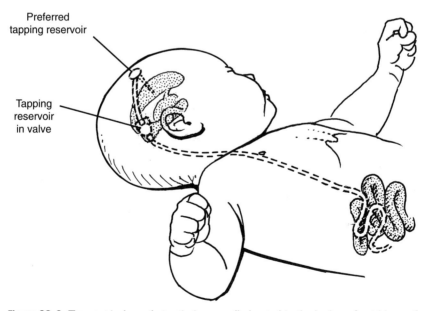

Preferred
tapping reservoir

Tapping
reservoir
in valve

Figure 38–2. The ventricular catheter tip is generally located in the body or frontal horn of
the ventricle. All catheters also contain a tapping reservoir, a pressure regulated valve, and
distal catheter.

    b. Valve
1. Virtually all shunts have a pressure-regulated valve to control cerebral spinal fluid (CSF) flow and to prevent excessive drainage.
2. Most valves are connected to the ventricular catheter by tubing and are located behind the ear. Some are located immediately adjacent to the ventricular catheter (Figs. 38-3, 38-4).
3. Although some valves have integral tapping chambers, they are generally not as easy to use as reservoirs (Fig. 38-5). If they are punctured, great care must be taken not to damage the control mechanism. Injection or withdrawal should be avoided unless previously agreed on with the pediatric neurosurgeon.
4. Pumping (i.e., depressing) the valve should be avoided unless previously discussed with the pediatric neurosurgeon. Each valve has its own "feel," and little information is generally obtained by pumping.
    c. Distal catheter
1. The valve is connected to a length of tubing that drains the CSF.
2. This catheter is usually in the peritoneum but may be in the pleural cavity or right atrium—other sites are rarely used (Fig. 38-2).
3. The tubing may exit the body and drain into a sterile closed-system collecting device (i.e., external ventriculostomy).
2. The most important aspect of the evaluation for shunt malfunction is the history provided by the patient. If the patient has symptoms of increased intracranial pressure, shunt malfunction is likely. Important symptoms include:
    a. Morning headache with nausea and vomiting (but not diarrhea or fever)
    b. Lethargy (not "napping too much")
    c. Pounding headache
    d. Intermittent headache with a crescendo pattern
    e. Headache that worsens with activity or later in the day and lessens in a reclining position suggests CSF overdrainage or a low pressure problem.
3. Physical examination findings may also contribute to the clinical diagnosis of shunt malfunction
    a. Head circumference—must compare to prior measurements
    b. Anterior fontanelle—size and fullness
    c. Funduscopy—children with myelomeningocele can have elevated intracranial pressure (ICP), which causes papilledema and blindness without headache.
    d. Mental status—level of consciousness and the patient's degree of comfort
4. The diagnostic studies that may assist in the determination of shunt function include
    a. Shunt radiograph series—to check for physical continuity of the shunt
    b. Head computed tomography (CT)—generally will need to compare this to prior studies. Note that some children with so-called slit ventricle syndrome do not get enlarged ventricles in spite of elevated ICP.
    c. Shunt tap—to measure ICP and to assess flow
    d. Shunt patency studies are used by some neurosurgeons but are not generally relied on, owing to a high false-negative result rate.
5. Occasionally, evaluation in the operating room is necessary to ascertain whether the shunt is operating properly.

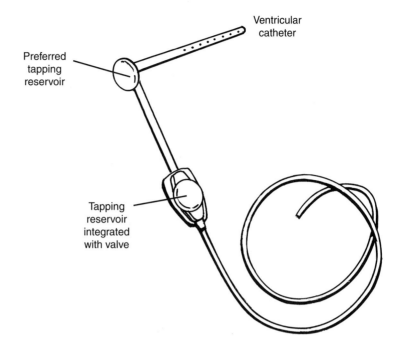

Figure 38–3. One example of a ventricular catheter with two reservoirs, one on the catheter and one on the valve. Here the preferred tapping reservoir is on the catheter.

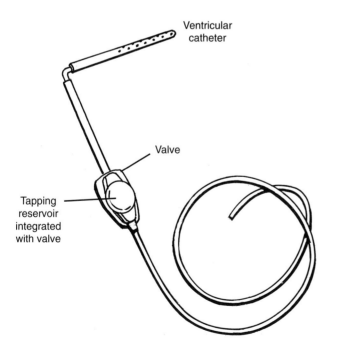

Figure 38–4. Example of a ventricular catheter with only one reservoir on the pressure regulating valve.

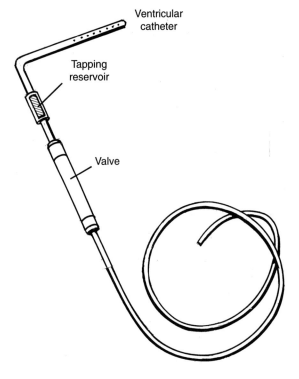

Ventricular catheter

Tapping reservoir

Valve

Figure 38–5. An example of a ventricular catheter in which the tapping mechanism is integral to the catheter. These are particularly easy to damage.

COMPLICATIONS

1. Inaccurate assessment of shunt function

References

McComb JG. Techniques for CSF diversion. In Scott M (ed). *Concepts in Neurosurgery,* Vol 3. Baltimore, Williams & Wilkins, 1990.
Post EM. Shunt systems. In Wilkins RH, Rengachary SS (eds). *Neurosurgery Update II.* New York, McGraw-Hill, 1991.
Scott RM. Shunt complications. In Wilkins RH, Rengachary SS (eds). *Neurosurgery Update II.* New York, McGraw-Hill, 1991.

CHAPTER 39

Timothy Mapstone and Patty Batchelder

VENTRICULAR SHUNT PUNCTURE

INDICATIONS

1. Assessing shunt function and to rule out elevated intracranial pressure
2. To obtain ventricular cerebral spinal fluid (CSF) for laboratory evaluation
3. To drain excessive ventricular CSF
4. For the injection of pharmacologic agents for therapy or diagnosis

CONTRAINDICATIONS

1. Local infection
2. Systemic infection
3. Marginal skin coverage (relative)
4. Subarachnoid CSF (as opposed to ventricular CSF) is required (e.g., to rule out meningitis)

EQUIPMENT

1. Small-bore (<23-gauge) or side-cutting Huber needle. (If Huber needle is not available, a needle with a stylet is preferred.)
2. Betadine solution
3. Manometer and 3-way stopcock
4. Tubes for CSF collection
5. 5–10 mg gentamicin in 1-ml volume
6. Two 3-cc syringes
7. Sterile normal saline for injection
8. Sterile gloves and towels, facemask
9. Razor
10. Collodion and sterile cottonball

CAUTION: Ventricular catheters are highly variable, and particular types can be difficult to identify on exterior examination. It is wise to discuss tapping with the neurosurgeon prior to the procedure. Some surgeons prefer to perform this procedure themselves.

PROCEDURE

1. Identify site of reservoir (Fig. 39-1). Shave a small patch of hair over the tapping reservoir.
2. Prep the shaved area with Betadine.
3. Puncture the reservoir with Huber needle (or needle and stylet) (Fig. 39-2).
4. Remove the stylet and observe for spontaneous CSF flow. Collect the amount needed for diagnostic studies.
5. *Do not withdraw* CSF unless it is *absolutely* certain that the ventricular catheter is completely surrounded by CSF and is not blocked.
6. If there is no free flow, and you are certain that the puncture was in a correct location, inject approximately 0.5 ml of sterile saline into the reservoir. Then remove the syringe and observe for flow. If there remains no flow, do not repeat the injection. Stop the procedure and notify the pediatric neurosurgeon.
7. When the procedure is complete, inject the gentamicin (5 mg for a body weight <3 kg and 10 mg for all others) into the ventricular catheter before withdrawing the needle (Fig. 39-3).
8. No dressing is required. If CSF droplets appear on the skin, seal the area with collodion and a sterile cottonball.

COMPLICATIONS

1. Infection
2. Laceration of the reservoir

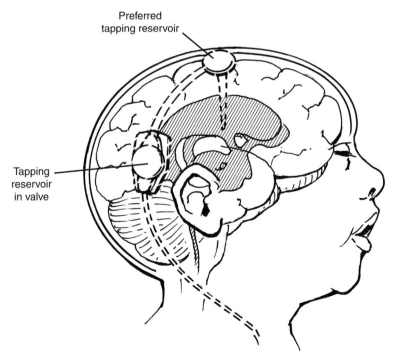

Figure 39–1. Close-up view of ventricular catheter in place. Tapping reservoirs are indicated.

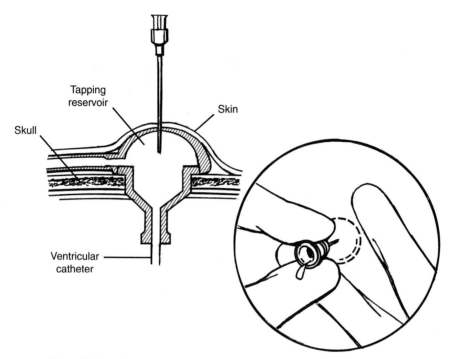

Skull

Tapping
reservoir

Skin

Ventricular
catheter

Figure 39–2. After preparation, the Huber needle is inserted into the reservoir.

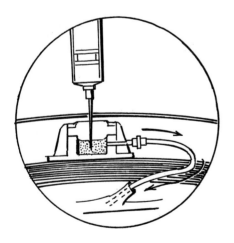

Figure 39–3. Gentamicin is injected after the procedure is completed.

3. Catheter occlusion secondary to efforts to withdraw CSF
4. Introduction of air into the vascular system if patient has ventricular-atrial shunt

References

McComb JG. Techniques for CSF Diversion. In Scott M (ed). *Concepts in Neurosurgery* (Vol 3). Baltimore, Williams & Wilkins, 1990.

Post EM. Shunt systems. In Wilkins RH, Rengachary SS (eds). *Neurosurgery Update II.* New York, McGraw-Hill, 1991.

Scott RM. Shunt complications. In Wilkins RH, Rengachary SS (eds). *Neurosurgery Update II.* New York, McGraw-Hill, 1991.

SOFT TISSUE AND WOUND REPAIR

CHAPTER 40

Steven Krug

REGIONAL NERVE BLOCKS

INDICATIONS

1. Local anesthesia of skin in area supplied by a sensory nerve

   Digital nerve—finger, toe, nailbed
   Radial nerve—dorsal aspect of the hand, thumb, and index and middle fingers
   Median nerve—palmar aspect of the hand (radial side), thumb, and index and middle fingers
   Ulnar nerve—dorsal and palmar ulnar aspects of the hand, fifth finger, and the ulnar aspect of the fourth finger
   Intercostal nerve—rib as well as the overlying skin in the thorax
   Supraorbital nerve—forehead and scalp above the eyes and the upper eyelid
   Infraorbital nerve—midface including upper lip, cheek, nose, and lower eyelid
   Mental nerve—lower face including the chin and lower lip

CONTRAINDICATIONS

   None

EQUIPMENT

1. Povidone-iodine solution
2. Syringe 3- to 5-cc
3. 25- or 27-gauge needle, 1 to 2 in
4. 1% lidocaine (without epinephrine) or 1% mepivacaine for longer procedures
5. 8.4% sodium bicarbonate—this may be mixed with the lidocaine in a 1:9 part ratio (1 part $NaHCO_3$ to 9 parts lidocaine) to reduce the pain associated with injection
6. Gloves

PROCEDURES

General Considerations

1. Carefully examine the area to be anesthetized for neurovascular function before injecting lidocaine.

2. Identify landmarks of injection site and prepare the skin with povidone-iodine solution.
3. Before intradermal injection of lidocaine, aspirate the syringe to avoid an intravascular injection.
4. Upon completion of injection, wait approximately 10 to 15 min for onset of anesthesia.

Digital Nerve

1. The digital nerves may be found on either side of the digit in both volar and dorsal locations. Anesthetic must be injected at all four nerves for a sufficient block.
2. Position the hand with the dorsal side down on a flat surface. Note that it may be necessary to immobilize the limb and the digit in an uncooperative patient.
3. Identify the needle insertion site on the dorsolateral aspect of the digit just distal to the metacarpophalangeal joint adjacent to the web space (Fig. 40-1A).
4. Insert the needle 2 to 3 mm at a 45-degree angle to a position just lateral to the bone and inject 0.5 to 1 ml of lidocaine (Fig. 40-1B).
5. Straighten and advance the needle deeper until it reaches the volar aspect of the bone, where another 0.5 to 1.0 ml of lidocaine will be injected (Fig. 40-1C).
6. Withdraw the needle and repeat the process on the other side of the digit.

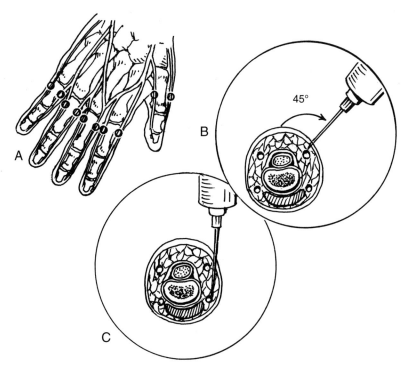

Figure 40–1. Digital nerve block. *A,* Needle insertion sites are indicated by solid circles. *B,* Insert needle into digit adjacent to dorsal branch of the digital nerve. *C,* Advance needle to inject adjacent to the ventral branch.

7. A similar result may be obtained by inserting the needle directly into the web space between the digits (Fig. 40-2) and injecting 1 to 2 ml of lidocaine.

8. Upon completion of injection, one should wait approximately 5 min for onset of anesthesia.

Radial Nerve

1. The sensory cutaneous branch of the radial nerve separates from the trunk of the radial nerve proximal to the wrist, and runs over the dorsal surface of the radial head near the radial styloid.

2. Palpating the radial styloid, begin the subcutaneous injection of lidocaine 2 to 4 cm proximal to the styloid (Fig. 40-3).

3. Inject a continuous subcutaneous wheal of lidocaine starting from the styloid medially over the dorsum of the hand to the lateral radial epicondyle. If these landmarks cannot be found, one can also use the lateral margin of the "anatomic snuffbox," the tendon of the extensor hallucis brevis, and the extensor carpi radialis tendon, as the lateral and medial markers for anesthetic infiltration (Fig. 40-3).

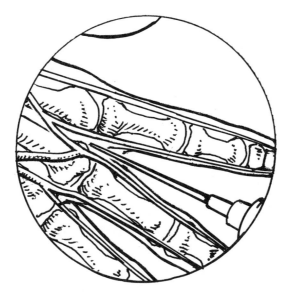

Figure 40–2. Needle insertion into web space.

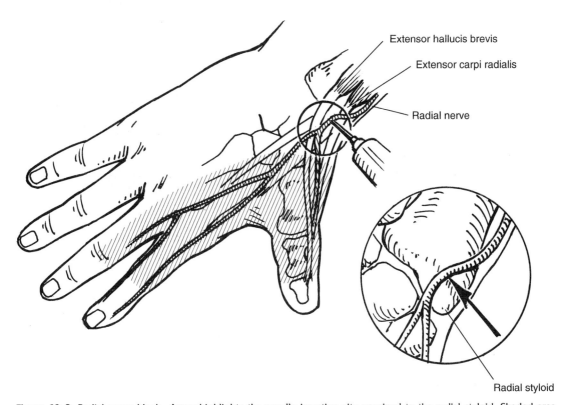

Extensor hallucis brevis

Extensor carpi radialis

Radial nerve

Radial styloid

Figure 40–3. Radial nerve block. *Arrow* highlights the needle insertion site proximal to the radial styloid. Shaded area represents the area of anesthesia.

Median Nerve

1. The median nerve may be located at the level of the proximal wrist crease between the tendons of the flexor carpi radialis and palmaris longus. Locating these tendons will be aided by having the patient make a fist and flex the wrist (Fig. 40-4).
2. Insert the needle over the nerve at the proximal crease and advance to a depth of 0.5 to 1 cm (Fig. 40-5). In older children, the presence of paresthesia ensures proper needle position.
3. Inject 3 ml of lidocaine and allow 5 to 10 min for onset of anesthesia. If paresthesia was not elicited, consider injection of 4 to 5 ml rather than 3 ml.

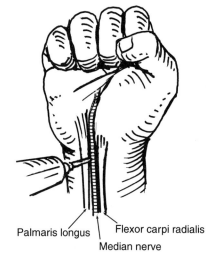

Figure 40–4. Median nerve block. Location of median nerve is at proximal wrist crease.

Palmaris longus | Flexor carpi radialis

Median nerve

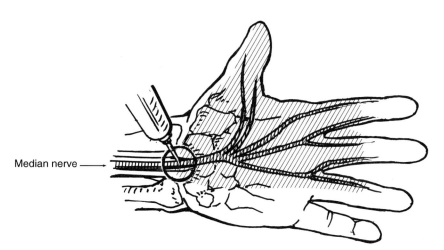

Median nerve

Figure 40–5. Needle insertion site for median nerve block. Shaded area represents the area of anesthesia.

Ulnar Nerve

1. The ulnar nerve may be blocked at the wrist or at the elbow. The ulnar nerve divides into two branches (palmar and dorsal) just proximal to the wrist. Wrist level blocks may be less successful owing to failure to anesthetize both branches.
2. At the wrist, inject an intradermal wheal of lidocaine over the ulnar nerve at the level of the proximal wrist crease and the ulnar styloid (Fig. 40-6). The nerve is typically located on the ulnar side of the ulnar artery and medial to the flexor carpi ulnaris tendon.
3. Advance the needle to a depth of 5 to 6 mm. This should provoke paresthesia. Inject 3 ml of lidocaine. If paresthesia was not elicited, inject 5 ml rather than 3 ml.
4. If the dorsal sensory branch (ulnar aspect of the palm) is not adequately blocked, this may be accomplished by injecting 2 to 3 ml of lidocaine subcutaneously on the dorsal surface just distal to the ulnar styloid.
5. At the elbow, the ulnar nerve may be located between the medial epicondyle and the olecranon. Flexing the elbow will assist in locating the nerve (Fig. 40-7).
6. Inject an intradermal wheal of lidocaine, using 3 to 5 ml. Take care not to inject directly into the nerve but rather on either side of the nerve. If paresthesia occurs, withdraw the needle 2 to 3 mm to avoid intraneural injection.

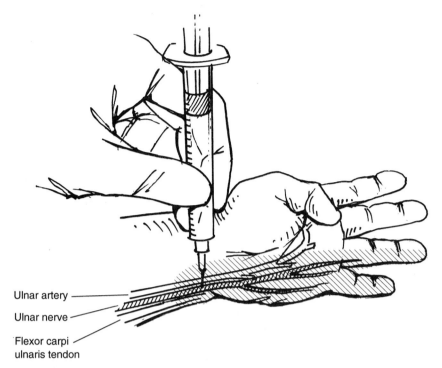

Ulnar artery

Ulnar nerve

Flexor carpi
ulnaris tendon

Figure 40–6. Ulnar nerve block. Insertion site is shown at the wrist. Shaded area represents the area of anesthesia.

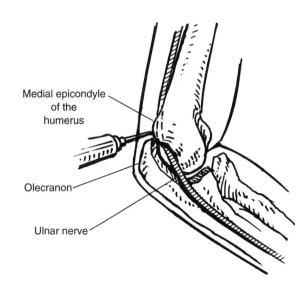

Figure 40–7. Insertion site for ulnar nerve block is at the elbow.

Medial epicondyle
of the
humerus

Olecranon

Ulnar nerve

Intercostal Nerve

1. Each thoracic nerve exits the spine at the intervertebral foramen. After splitting off a posterior cutaneous nerve, it runs along the inferior border of the rib in the subcostal groove, giving off lateral cutaneous branches at the midaxillary line. These branches provide sensory function for the anterior and lateral chest wall.
2. Nerve blocks are usually performed between the posterior axillary and the midaxillary line, or at a point proximal to the branching of the lateral cutaneous nerve.
3. The index finger of the nondominant hand should be placed at the chosen site of injection and used to retract the skin overlying the rib in a cephalad direction.
4. The needle is then inserted at an 80-degree angle pointing cephalad at the tip of the finger that is retracting the skin over the rib. The hand holding the needle should rest on the chest to allow for additional stability and safety. The needle should then be advanced until it meets with the lower margin of the rib (Fig. 40-8A).
5. The retracted skin should then be released. This will serve to position the needle at a 90-degree angle with the position of the needle tip at the inferior border of the rib (Fig. 40-8B).
6. The needle should then be "walked" down the surface of the rib until the superior border of the intercostal space is found. Carefully advance the needle 2 to 3 mm and inject 1 to 5 ml of lidocaine (Fig. 40-8C).
7. To allow for cross-innervation, the procedure should be repeated for the rib above and the rib below.

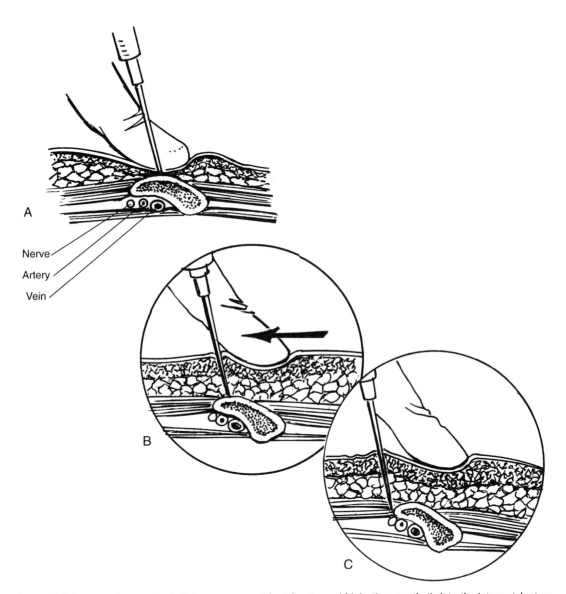

Nerve

Artery

Vein

Figure 40–8. Intercostal nerve block. Extreme care must be taken to avoid injecting anesthetic into the intercostal artery, which is adjacent to the nerve.

Supraorbital Nerve

1. The supraorbital nerve exits the skull at the foramen located on the medial aspect of the supraorbital ridge (Fig. 40-9).
2. Palpating the foramen, insert the needle just medial to the foramen and advance toward the foramen to a depth of approximately 0.5 to 1 cm (Fig. 40-10). In older children, the presence of paresthesia ensures proper needle position.
3. Inject 1 to 3 ml of lidocaine. Allow 5 min for onset of anesthesia.

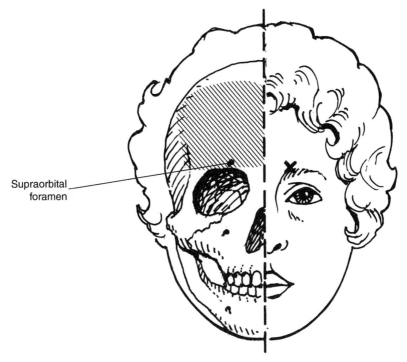

Supraorbital
foramen

Figure 40–9. Supraorbital nerve block. Insert needle at the X. Shaded area indicates area of ipsilateral anesthesia.

Figure 40–10. Insert needle into foramina located on medial aspect of supraorbital ridge.

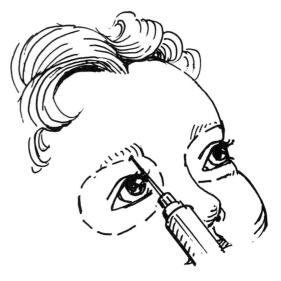

Infraorbital Nerve

1. The infraorbital nerve exits the skull at the foramen located inferior to the medial aspect of the infraorbital ridge (Fig. 40-11). This is best accessed from inside the mouth.
2. With the thumb and index finger of the nondominant hand lifting the upper lip, and with the middle finger palpating the foramen, insert the needle at the upper gum line along the axis of the second upper bicuspid (Fig. 40-12).
3. Advance the needle until it is felt at the level of the foramen (2 to 6 cm, depending on the patient's age) and inject 1 to 2 ml of lidocaine. Wait 5 min for onset of anesthesia.

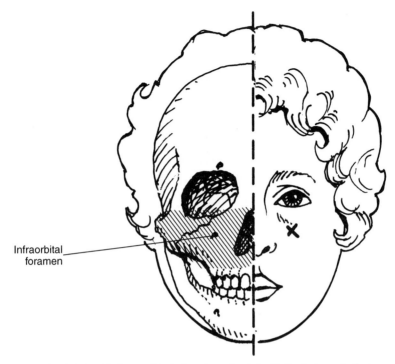

Infraorbital
foramen

Figure 40–11. Infraorbital nerve block. Insert needle at the X. Shaded area indicates the area of ipsilateral anesthesia.

Figure 40–12. The infraorbital nerve is best accessed from inside the mouth. The needle is inserted into the foramina, which may be palpated at the upper gum line.

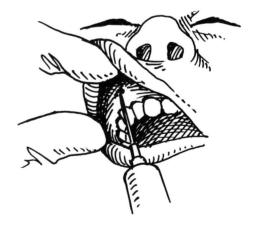

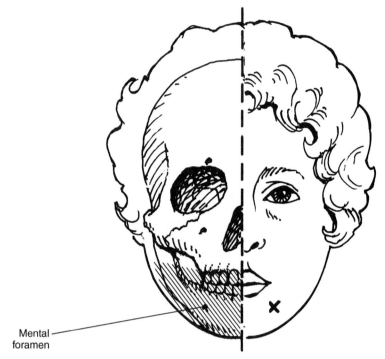

Mental
foramen

Figure 40–13. Mental nerve block. Insert needle at the X. Shaded area indicates the area of ipsilateral anesthesia.

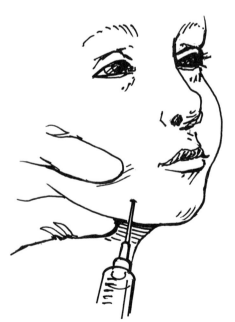

Figure 40–14. The mental nerve may be located at the foramen, which typically lies in a straight line with the supraorbital and infraorbital foramina.

Mental Nerve

1. The mental nerve exits the mandible at the foramen located on its lateromedial aspect at the level of the premolar. This foramen typically lies in a straight line with the supraorbital and infraorbital foramina (Fig. 40-13).
2. Palpating the foramen, insert the needle just medial to the foramen, advancing 0.5 to 1 cm toward the foramen (Fig. 40-14). In older children, the presence of paresthesia ensures proper needle position.
3. Inject 1 to 2 ml of lidocaine. Allow 5 min for onset of anesthesia.

COMPLICATIONS

1. Infection
2. Hemorrhage
3. Intravascular injection
4. Intraneural injection and postoperative anesthesia
5. Intra-articular injection
6. Pneumothorax or hemothorax (intercostal)

References

Amsterdam J. Regional anesthesia of the head and neck. In Roberts JR, Hedges JR (eds). *Clinical Procedures in Emergency Medicine* (2nd ed). Philadelphia, WB Saunders, 1991.

Butterworth JF. *Atlas of Procedures in Anesthesia and Critical Care.* Philadelphia, WB Saunders, 1992.

Orlinsky M, Dean E. Local and topical anesthesia and nerve blocks of the thorax and extremities. In Roberts JR, Hedges JR (eds). *Clinical Procedures in Emergency Medicine* (2nd ed). Philadelphia, WB Saunders, 1991.

Ruddy RM (ed). Illustrated techniques of pediatric emergency procedures. In Fleisher GR, Ludwig S (eds). *Textbook of Pediatric Emergency Medicine* (3rd ed). Baltimore, Williams & Wilkins, 1993.

CHAPTER 41

Cynthia Hoecker

SIMPLE SUTURING

INDICATIONS

1. Closure of uncomplicated lacerations

RELATIVE CONTRAINDICATIONS

1. Heavily contaminated wounds or clean wounds more than 12 to 24 hr old
2. Most bite wounds (especially nonfacial)
3. High-velocity missile injuries
4. Complex crush injuries

EQUIPMENT

1. Sterile 0.9% saline for irrigation (1 liter)
2. 10% Betadine solution
3. Tissue forceps (toothed preferable)
4. Needle holder
5. Suture/iris scissors
6. Hemostats
7. Scalpel #15 blade (if removal of devitalized tissue necessary)
8. 30-cc syringe for irrigation (splash guard attachment optional)
9. Angiocatheter attached to irrigating syringe to help direct stream and provide higher pressure irrigation
10. Suture material (Tables 41–1, 41–2, and 41–3) with ½- to ⅜-circle conventional cutting (▲) or reverse cutting (▼) needle
11. Sterile basin
12. Local anesthetic
13. 8.4% sodium bicarbonate solution (for buffering lidocaine)
14. 3- to 5-cc syringe (for local anesthetic) with small-gauge (25-30) needle
15. Sterile sponges
16. Sterile towels
17. Sterile gloves, protective eyewear, mask, gown (optional)

Table 41-1. COMMONLY USED SUTURE MATERIAL FOR EMERGENCY WOUND REPAIR

	Content	Characteristics	Uses	Tensile Strength	Tissue Reactivity
Nonabsorbable					
Nylon (Ethilon, Dermalon)	Monofilament nylon	"Memory"—decreased knot security (4–5 throws required)	Percutaneous closures Common facial suture	Good Maintained >1 yr	Minimal
Polypropylene (Prolene)	Monofilament polymer of propylene	"Memory"—decreased knot security	Percutaneous closures Facial and skin closures Pull-out dermal closures	Excellent	Less reactive than nylon
Silk	Derived from protein made by silkworm larvae	Good knot security Superior handling qualities Increased infection risk Behaves as a very slowly absorbed suture Multifilament/braided	Limited in emergency wound care Potential use for oral mucosal repairs	Good (lost after 1 yr)	Highly reactive; tissue ingrowth therefore difficult and painful suture removal
Absorbable					
Plain gut	Collagen from sheep intestines Monofilament	High tendency to fray Stiff Absorption time 7–10 d	Ligating vessels Subcutaneous Mucosal surfaces	Maintained 7–10 d	Highly tissue reactive
Chromic gut	Gut treated with chromium salts to delay absorption	Absorption time 15–90 d (7–10 d oral cavity)	Oral cavity Fascia	Maintained 10–14 d (7–10 d in oral cavity) Stronger than plain gut	Highly tissue reactive
Fast-absorbing gut	Heat-treated gut	Absorption time 5–7 d	Epidermal suturing when sutures needed <1 wk	5–7 d until absorption Less strength than plain gut	Highly tissue reactive
Polyglactin 910 (Vicryl)	Copolymer of lactide and glycolide	Multifilament, braided Absorption 40–90 d Hydrolyzed	Subcutaneous sutures	Maintains 60% tensile strength at 14 d	Less than gut
Polydioxanone (PDS)	Polydioxanone monofilament	Synthetic Low-friction coefficient Hydrolyzed in vivo	Extended wound support	Minimal absorption until 90 d	Minimal tissue reactivity
Polyglycolic acid (PGA) (Dexon)	Homopolymer of glycolic acid	Multifilament, braided Absorption—120 d (16–20 d oral cavity) High tissue drag	Subcutaneous closures Vessel ligation	Maintained up to 120 d	Less reactive than gut

d = days.

Table 41–2. **BASIC GUIDE TO SUTURE CHOICE**

Location	Suture Type	Size
Skin	Nylon or polypropylene	4-0 (extremity, torso); 5-0 (hand),
	Fast-absorbing gut (face only)	6-0 (face)
Mucous membranes	Chromic gut	4-0, 5-0
Subcutaneous	Vicryl, Dexon	4-0, 5-0

PROCEDURE

1. History. Ascertain the time and mechanism of injury as well as the underlying health status of the patient, including a history of medications, allergies, and tetanus immunization.
2. Physical examination. After donning protective wear, perform a neurovascular examination and an examination of musculotendinous function of anatomic structures potentially affected by the laceration.
3. Initial cleansing. With the patient in a relaxed position, cleanse the skin adjacent to the wound with normal saline (in nonmucous membrane locations Betadine solution may be added). Generally, 1 part 10% Betadine solution should be added to 9 parts sterile saline to generate a 1% Betadine solution.
4. Analgesia
   a. Lidocaine 1%. This is the most commonly used local anesthetic agent in emergency wound care. The addition of epinephrine to decrease local bleeding is optional but is strictly contraindicated for use on distal extremities (e.g., digits, penis, pinna, tip of nose). Buffering lidocaine with 8.4% sodium bicarbonate using a 9:1 ratio (9 parts lidocaine to 1 part bicarbonate) reduces the pain of injection. Infiltrate the wound margins with the anesthetic solution using a small- (25–30) gauge needle taking care to draw back on the syringe before injection to avoid injecting into a vessel. The maximum recommended dose of lidocaine in children is 5 mg/kg for lidocaine alone or 7 mg/kg for lidocaine with epinephrine.
   b. TAC. This is a combination local anesthetic that can be applied topically to minor lacerations on the face and scalp. Generally the solution is composed

Table 41–3. **BASIC GUIDE TO NEEDLE CHOICE**

Needle Type	Cross Section	Characteristics	Designation	Tissue Use
Conventional Cutting	(▲)	3 cutting edges with an inside cutting edge—greater tendency to cut through the tissue edge than the reverse cutting needle	PC* CPS	Skin
Reverse Cutting	(▼)	3 cutting edges with an outside cutting edge—most commonly used needle for skin closures; least traumatic to tissues	P* PS* FS CP PRE* SBE CE	Skin
Round/Tapered Point	(●)	No cutting edges; more difficult to hold with needle holders; appropriate for fascia, muscle, tendon closures		Fascia, muscle, tendon

*P, PS, PC, PRE—designation of plastic grade needles (needletip honed more sharply)

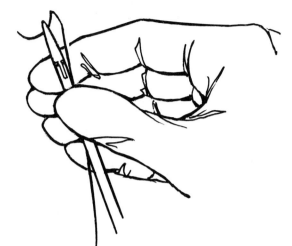

Figure 41–1. Load the needle holder.

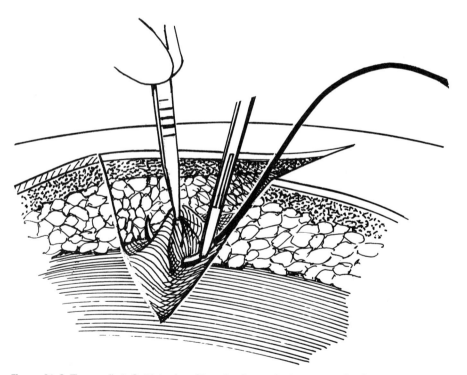

Figure 41–2. The needle is first introduced into the deeper fascia on one side of the wound, exiting in a more superficial position in the dermis.

of 1% tetracaine, 1:2000 epinephrine, and between 4 and 11.8% cocaine. The smaller concentration of cocaine is safer as rare cases of systemic toxicity have been reported owing to cocaine toxicity from TAC use. Saturate a cotton-tipped applicator or cottonball with 1 to 2 ml of TAC solution and apply directly to the laceration for 10 to 15 min. Care should be taken to ensure that there is no contact of the solution with the mucous membranes of the eyes, mouth, or nose. There should be a circumferential area of blanching around the laceration site when anesthetized. Test the area of adequacy of analgesia using a needletip and supplement with additional local anesthetic (TAC or lidocaine) until the patient can be comfortably sutured.

   c. Lidocaine/Epinephrine/Tetracaine (LET). This is a combination topical anesthetic composed of 4% lidocaine, 1:1000 epinephrine, and 1% tetracaine. It has been demonstrated to provide a level of local anesthesia comparable to that achieved with TAC. It is applied in a similar fashion to that of TAC.

5. Debridement. After the wound has been adequately anesthetized, debride or incise nonviable or contaminated tissue at the wound margins, using scissors or scalpel if necessary.

6. Irrigation. Irrigate the wound well with saline solution using high-pressure irrigation. This may be achieved by attaching a 19-gauge or smaller angiocatheter to the irrigating syringe. Maximum irrigating pressures as high as 50 psi may be safely used in cases of heavy contamination using pulsatile jet flow devices (e.g., Water Pik). Several hundred milliliters to 1 liter of irrigant is generally required, depending on the wound size and degree of contamination. Try to avoid scrubbing tissues. There should be no debris visible in the wound when finished with the step.

7. Preparation of a sterile field. Once the wound has been adequately cleansed, prepare the area around the wound using Betadine solution. (Betadine should not be applied to mucous membranes.) Drape the area with sterile towels until a limited sterile surgical field is obtained.

8. Exploration. Explore the wound using a sterile gloved finger to identify the depth and extent of injury to important underlying structures (e.g., skull fracture or galeal disruption under a scalp laceration).

9. Planning the closure. Identify which structures in addition to the skin surface will need reapproximation (e.g., fascia or subcutaneous tissue) in order to eliminate dead space or to decrease tension at the surface wound edges. Choose the appropriate suture type(s) and have it placed on the sterile tray (Tables 41-1, 41-2, and 41-3).

10. Loading the needle. Load the needle onto the needle holder with the needle held approximately one third of the way from the swage end. The needle should be at a 90-degree angle relative to the needle holder (Fig. 41-1).

11. Deep closure. For deep or gaping wounds, begin reapproximation with the deepest tissues (fascia and subcutaneous tissue) first. If layered closure is necessary, it is important to employ a technique that will "bury" the knot. The needle is first introduced into one side of the wound, entering the deeper superficial fascia and exiting in the dermis (Fig. 41-2). The use of tissue forceps will be necessary to gently pull up on and expose the tissues while a "bite" is being taken. The needle is then introduced into the dermis on other side of the wound, exiting in the superficial fascia (Fig. 41-3). As the leading and trailing ends of the suture are now on the same or inferior side of the suture loop, the knot, when tied, will be buried (Fig. 41-4).

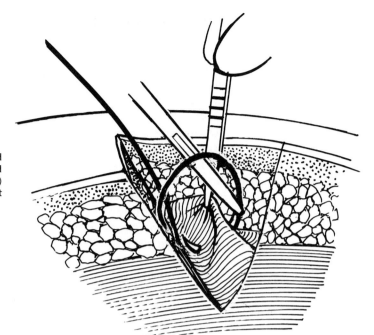

Figure 41–3. The needle is passed through the opposite side of the wound in a direction (i.e., superficial to deep) that is opposite that used on the first side.

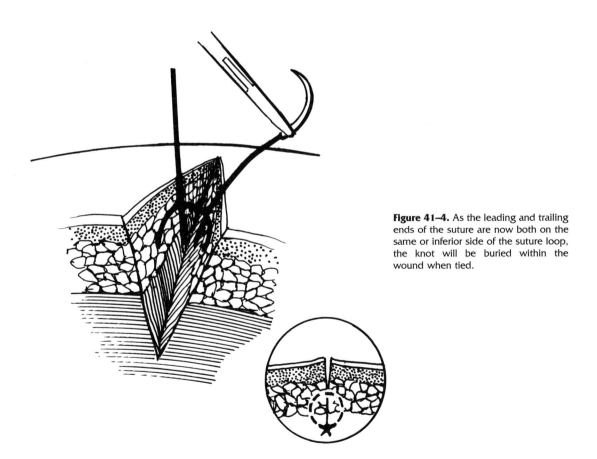

Figure 41–4. As the leading and trailing ends of the suture are now both on the same or inferior side of the suture loop, the knot will be buried within the wound when tied.

12. Skin closure. When approximating the skin surface it is desirable to attain slightly everted wound edges. This is accomplished by entering the skin with the needle at an angle of 90 degrees and driving the needle tip downward and slightly outward to follow a circular pathway (Fig. 41-5). As the needle completes its circular course, the tip should become visible on the opposite side of the laceration from needle entry at a point equidistant from the wound margin (Fig. 41-5). This technique for a simple interrupted suture may be accomplished with a single supinating motion of the wrist. Other types of stitches (the horizontal and vertical mattress) are described later.

13. Tying the knot. Securing the suture is accomplished by performing an instrument tie and a surgeon's knot (Fig. 41-6). This knot has a double first throw to allow for added knot security and can be used for both deep and superficial closures. The second throw forms a square knot with the first. Generally four to five throws are necessary to fully secure a suture. Be careful not to tie the knot too tightly, as this can impair blood flow and wound healing.

14. Completing the closure. Subsequent stitches are placed in a similar manner, using as few stitches as possible to adequately approximate wound edges without gaps. Knots should be placed to one side or the other of the wound.

15. Aftercare
    a. Cleansing. Following wound closure, clean away blood on the skin surface.
    b. Dressing. Most wounds benefit from a clean, dry protective dressing to protect and absorb drainage. An exception to this is small scalp wounds, which are difficult to dress. The exact type of dressing used will depend on the size and location of the wound and may range from a single Band-Aid to splint-immobilization (wound overlying a joint). The benefit of applying antibiotic ointments (e.g., Neosporin, bacitracin) to the freshly sutured wound has not been well proven; however, this practice does decrease the adherence of the wound to the dressing material. A nonadherent material (e.g., Adaptic) can serve the same purpose.

16. Suture removal. Sutures should be removed after a sufficient amount of time has elapsed to allow for the initial phases of wound healing. The amount of time needed depends on wound location, rate of healing (host factors), and degree of tension on the wound. For a guide to the recommended schedule for suture removal, see Table 41-4. The procedure for suture removal entails the use of tissue forceps and a sharp pair of scissors. The suture end, or tag, is grasped by the tissue forceps and gently pulled away from the skin until a scissor can be inserted under the loop of the suture and cut. Hydrogen peroxide solution can be used to dissolve dried blood from the wound edge, if needed, to locate and expose suture ends.

Table 41–4. **TIME TO SUTURE REMOVAL**

Location	Suture Removal
Face	3–5 days
Scalp	5–10 days
Trunk/Extremities	7–14 days

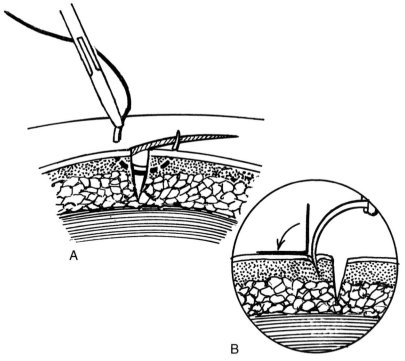

Figure 41–5. The needle should enter the skin at a 90-degree angle. It should be inserted in a manner that allows it to follow a circular course. For small wounds, the tip should become visible on the opposite side of the wound from the entry site.

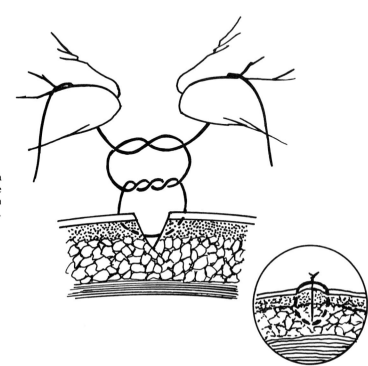

Figure 41–6. The surgeon's knot, a double first throw followed by a single second throw, will help to maintain the integrity of the suture as it is tied.

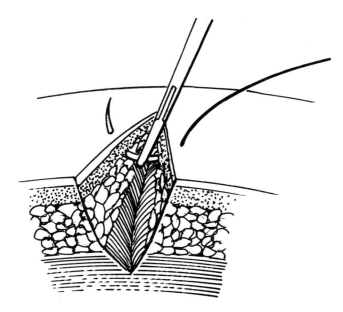

Figure 41–9. The interrupted horizontal stitch begins much like a simple interrupted stitch, entering and exiting the wound between 0.5 and 1 cm from the wound edge.

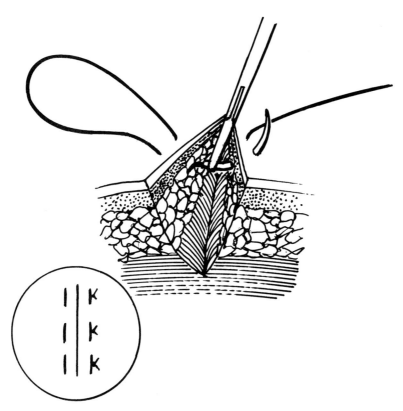

Figure 41–10. On the second pass of the interrupted horizontal stitch, the wound is reentered approximately 0.5 cm lateral or medial to the first exit site. The needle should exit the wound at a distance from the wound edge and trailing end of the suture similar to that used on entry.

Interrupted Horizontal Mattress Stitch

1. The horizontal mattress stitch provides good wound edge eversion and saves time, compared with performing a series of simple interrupted stitches. It can be used to help attain good wound edge eversion in areas of tissue laxity or on flexural surfaces (e.g., knee or elbow), where tissue edges tend to fold inward.
2. After following previous steps 1 through 11, the needle is passed through the tissue as if performing a simple interrupted stitch (Fig. 41-9).
3. Instead of tying the knot, the needle is loaded on the holder in the opposite direction and another pass through the tissue edges is made. This second bite is taken approximately 0.5 cm adjacent (lateral or medial) to the first exit site, and exits the other side of the wound, also one-half centimeter from the original entry site (Fig. 41-10).
4. The two ends are then tied using the surgeon's knot described previously on the same side of the wound margins.

COMPLICATIONS OF WOUND CLOSURE

1. Wound infection
2. Wound dehiscence
3. Allergy to latex, iodine, or anesthetic agents
4. Ischemia or toxicity caused by injection of anesthetic directly into a vessel
5. Systemic toxicity from local anesthetic agents

References

Bernstein G. Needle basics. J Dermatol Surg Oncol 11:1177-1178, 1985.
Macht SD, et al. Sutures and suturing—Current concepts. J Oral Surg 26:710-712, 1978.
Markovchick V. Suture materials and mechanical after care. Emerg Med Clin North Am 4:673-689, 1992.
Moy RL, et al. A review of sutures and suturing techniques. J Dermatol Surg Onc 18:785-795, 1992.
Roberts JR, Hedges JR. *Clinical Procedures in Emergency Medicine,* (2nd ed). Philadelphia, WB Saunders, 1991, pp 515-565.
Swanson NA, et al. Suture materials, 1980s: Properties, uses and abuses. Int J Dermatol 21:373-378, 1982.
Trott A. *Wounds and Lacerations: Emergency Care and Closure.* St. Louis, Mosby-Year Book, 1991, pp 66-79, 96-121, 275-308.
Wallace WR, et al. Comparison of polyglycolic acid suture to black silk, chromic, and plain catgut in human oral tissues. J Oral Surg 28:739-745, 1970.

CHAPTER 42

Cynthia Hoecker

INCISION AND DRAINAGE OF A SIMPLE SKIN ABSCESS

INDICATIONS

Surgical incision followed by drainage is the treatment of choice for simple localized skin abscess (a fluctuant and tender collection of pus beneath the skin surface). Many nonfacial superficial skin abscesses are easily and safely treated in the emergency department on an outpatient basis. Consider consulting a specialist for facial, hand, deep, or anatomically complex abscesses.

CONTRAINDICATIONS

The emergency physician should strongly consider involving a specialist in the early treatment of anatomically complex (owing to extent or location) or high-risk abscesses (e.g., involving deep tissues, the hand, or the face). Facial abscesses are probably best treated by a plastic surgeon. Furthermore, treatment in the operating room should be considered for patients requiring a lengthy or painful procedure that cannot be done comfortably in the emergency department.

EVALUATION

Before the procedure, a complete history should be obtained to determine the likelihood of the presence of a foreign body, the patient's tetanus status, and the presence of any important underlying conditions or allergies. X-ray examinations may be necessary to help locate a radiopaque foreign body or to evaluate the underlying bone for evidence of osteomyelitis.

EQUIPMENT

1. Sterile drapes or towels
2. Sterile syringe and 25-gauge needle (for lidocaine administration)
3. Lidocaine 1 to 2% solution with or without epinephrine (for local analgesia)
4. Betadine solution
5. Sterile 4×4 gauze and other dressing supplies
6. Sterile scalpel, #11 blade
7. Sterile packing material (iodoform impregnated gauze is commonly used and is available in a variety of sizes)
8. One pair curved hemostats
9. Tissue forceps

PROCEDURE

1. Infiltrate the dermal tissues overlying the abscess with 1 to 2% lidocaine solution in a linear distribution approximating the line of incision (choose a line parallel to Langer's lines for cosmesis). If possible, a nerve block (e.g., digital block) should be used instead because of difficulty in obtaining optimal anesthesia by local infiltration of the skin overlying the abscess cavity.
2. Following anesthetization, prepare the skin over the abscess using Betadine scrub. Place sterile drapes over and around the site to obtain a limited sterile field.
3. Using the #11 scalpel blade, make a linear incision through the skin over the full length of the abscess cavity (Fig. 42-1A). Do not "stab" the tissue, but carefully incise. Be careful to avoid important neurovascular structures that may be nearby depending on the abscess location. If you are unfamiliar with the local anatomy or if the abscess is more than superficial, the procedure is best performed by a specialist (general or plastic surgeon).
4. Allow the pus to drain from the cavity. Using a sterile gloved finger or hemostats, explore the cavity and break up any loculations of pus (Fig. 42-1B). Mechanical suction using a sterile catheter can be used to aid pus drainage from a sizable cavity.

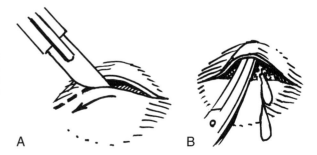

Figure 42–1. *A,* Make a linear incision through the skin over the full length of the abscess cavity. Pay careful attention to avoid adjacent neurovascular structures. *B,* Explore and drain the abscess cavity with a hemostat.

A   B

5. Place sterile packing material (or gauze in large cavities) inside the wound. The technique can be aided by the use of a blunt-ended hemostat or forceps used in the operator's dominant hand to gently pack the material into the cavity. Packing should fill the abscess cavity but not be packed so tightly as to threaten the blood supply. An end should be left hanging out of the incision so that it may be easily removed. The packing facilitates continued drainage of pus and fluid, prevents premature closure of the abscess cavity, and, upon removal, aids debridement.

6. A dry absorbent gauze dressing should be applied over the wound site. A secure, but not tight, circumferential dressing is preferable on extremities.

7. The first dressing change should occur in 24 to 48 hr, at which time the dressing and packing are removed. The wound is inspected for reaccumulation of pus or loculations and sometimes reanesthetized if further debridement or painful probing of the wound is needed.

8. The wound is repacked with a fresh packing and a new dressing is applied. The patient or parent should be instructed in the packing and dressing of the wound so that this can be done at home on a daily basis. After a few days, the patient can begin warm soaks or irrigation of the wound in the shower before the packing is replaced or the dressing reapplied. The wound should be rechecked by medical personnel every few days or more frequently if complications develop. Eventually the wound can be treated with warm soaks and dry dressings alone and allowed to heal by secondary intention.

9. Antibiotics are frequently prescribed but are arguably unnecessary for the treatment of uncomplicated abscesses that have been adequately drained in the immunocompetent host without a risk of endocarditis. The agents used should be directed against the most likely pathogens, usually pyogenic staphylococci, streptococci, and anaerobes.

COMPLICATIONS

1. Local spread of infection
2. Bacteremia and septicemia
3. Bleeding
4. Injury to nerves or vessels

References

Brook I, Finegold S. Aerobic and anaerobic bacteriology of cutaneous abscesses in children. Pediatrics 67(6):891–895, 1981.

Llera J, Levy R. Treatment of cutaneous abscess: A double-blind study. Ann Emerg Med 14(1):15–19, 1985.

Meislin H. Cutaneous abscesses—Anaerobic and aerobic bacteriology and outpatient management. Ann Intern Med 87(2):145–149, 1977.

Roberts JR, Hedges JR. *Clinical Procedures in Emergency Medicine* (2nd ed). Philadelphia, WB Saunders, 1991, pp 591–598.

CHAPTER 43

Cynthia Hoecker

INCISION AND DRAINAGE OF A PARONYCHIA

INDICATIONS

Paronychia, a common childhood condition, is an area of cellulitis adjacent to the nail plate that frequently leads to the accumulation of purulent material. If a pus-filled space exists, the proper treatment is drainage. The optimal mode of drainage depends on the location of the pus, which may be located under the nail (subungual), under the eponychium or cuticle (subeponychial), or a combination of these.

CONTRAINDICATIONS

There are no contraindications to drainage, which is the definitive treatment. Be aware of any underlying conditions (e.g., immunocompromised state or diabetes mellitus), which may complicate the healing process or indicate a need for inpatient treatment or closer outpatient follow-up.

EVALUATION

As for all procedures, it is important to ascertain the underlying health status of the patient, allergies, and tetanus status before beginning the procedure. The procedure, including the anesthetic plan, should be explained to the parent and patient.

EQUIPMENT

1. Sterile #11 scalpel
2. Betadine solution
3. Alcohol pads
4. Sterile towels and drapes
5. 1% lidocaine *without* epinephrine (for digital block)
6. 25-gauge needle (for digital block)
7. Sterile gauze
8. Rubber band (for use as a finger tourniquet)
9. Sterile gauze bandage

10. Sterile packing material (in case of nail root removal), iris scissors (if nail removal is necessary), sterile nonadherent mesh (possibly used as a stent between eponychium and germinal matrix when packing not used for this purpose), small straight hemostats

PROCEDURE

1. If any portion of the nail is to be removed or any skin incision made, a digital block should be performed before the procedure. If necessary, refer to the outline of the procedure for a digital block. (See Chapter 40.)
2. Once the finger is adequately anesthetized, prepare a limited sterile field, using the Betadine solution as a prep and sterile towels. A tourniquet can be placed at the base of the digit to decrease bleeding.
3. The drainage procedure depends on the type and extent of the paronychia.
   a. Simple paronychia: A simple paronychia is present if the collection of pus is limited to the area around the eponychium but not extending underneath the nail root or nail. This can be drained by simply placing the scalpel blade between the (eponychium) and the nail, allowing drainage of the purulent material (Fig. 43-1). In the case of a horseshoe paronychia this incision may need to be extended the length of the base of the nail.
   b. Complex paronychia: A more complicated situation exists when pus is present underneath the nail plate. Treatment of this condition necessitates partial removal of the nail overlying the pus. The nail plate is loose over the collection of pus and can usually be easily removed. An incision may need to be made into the skin overlying the nail root in order to expose it and allow cutting the proximal portion of the nail plate away using iris scissors (Fig. 43-2). A packing or stent must be placed to prevent the eponychium from scarring down and adhering to the germinal matrix and preventing proper nail regrowth.

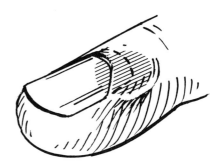

Figure 43-1. Method for drainage of a simple paronychia (see text).

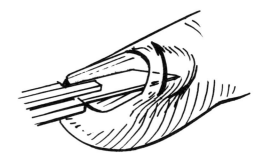

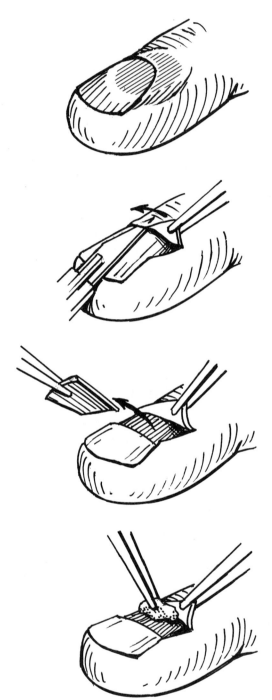

Figure 43–2. Drainage of a complex paronychia requires partial removal of the nail.

4. Following the drainage procedure, nail removal, and placement of packing or stent, a sterile bandage is applied to soak any continued drainage and to protect the wound. A Band-Aid can act as a dressing if a simple paronychia was drained.
5. Follow-up should occur in 24 to 48 hr, when the dressing is changed and the packing, if present, is replaced. The packing will no longer be necessary after about 1 wk and the patient can begin daily warm soaks and use a Band-Aid as a dressing. If no packing is placed, the patient can begin daily warm water soaks in the first 24 hr.
6. Antibiotics should be considered in all cases but are probably not necessary following drainage of a simple paronychia. Most paronychias are colonized with a mixture of aerobes (staphylococci and streptococci) and anaerobes.

COMPLICATIONS

1. Injury to neurovascular bundle (distal digital nerve and artery)
2. Improper regrowth of nail
3. Bacteremia
4. Increasing cellulitis following the procedure
5. Bleeding

References

Brook I. Aerobic and anaerobic microbiology of paronychia. Ann Emerg Med 19(9):994-996, 1990.
Hausman MR, Lisser SP. Hand infections. Orthop Clin North Am 23(1):171-185, 1992.
Roberts JR, Hedges JR. *Clinical Procedures in Emergency Medicine* (2nd ed). Philadelphia, WB Saunders, 1991, pp 604-605.
Trott A. *Wounds and Lacerations: Emergency Care and Closure.* St. Louis, Mosby–Year Book, 1991, pp 207-210.

CHAPTER 44

Cynthia Hoecker

INCISION AND DRAINAGE OF A FELON

INDICATIONS

A felon is an infection characterized by a collection of pus in the pulp space of the fingertip (Fig. 44-1). Drainage is the treatment of choice. Several methods of drainage have been described, but the most frequently used procedure will be described here.

CONTRAINDICATIONS

There are no contraindications to drainage, which is the definitive treatment. Be aware of any underlying conditions (e.g., immunocompromised state or diabetes mellitus) that may complicate the healing process or indicate a need for inpatient treatment or closer outpatient follow-up.

EVALUATION

As for all procedures, it is important to ascertain the underlying health status of the patient, allergies, and tetanus status before beginning the procedure. The procedure and anesthetic plan should be explained to the parent and patient before beginning.

EQUIPMENT

1. 1% Lidocaine *without* epinephrine (for digital block)
2. 25-gauge needle (digital block)
3. Sterile alcohol pads
4. Betadine solution
5. Sterile drapes or towels
6. Scalpel blade #11
7. Sterile gauze
8. Sterile drain (Penrose) or gauze (for packing wound)
9. Rubber band (for use as a finger tourniquet)

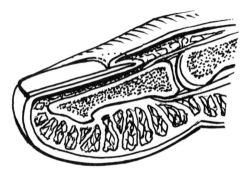

Figure 44–1. Cross-section of a digit demonstrates pulp space adjacent to distal phalanx.

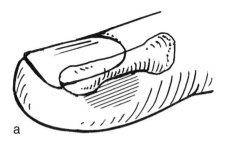

a

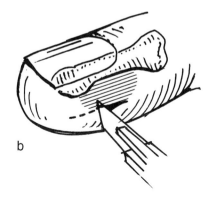

b

Figure 44–2. *A*, Purulent material localized in the pulp space volar to the distal phalanx. *B*, A longitudinal incision is made over the area of greatest fluctuance. *C*, After purulent material has drained partially, packing material is inserted to allow continued drainage.

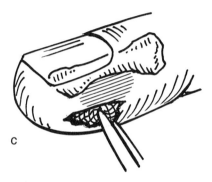

c

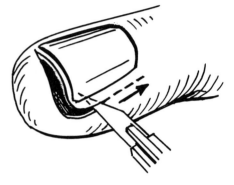

Figure 44–3. The hockey stick incision is to be used only for particularly extensive infections.

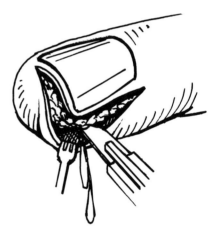

PROCEDURE

1. Perform a digital block on the involved finger. (See Chapter 40.)
2. Once the finger is adequately anesthetized, prepared a limited sterile field using the Betadine solution as a prep and sterile towels. A tourniquet can be placed at the base of the finger to decrease bleeding into the field.
3. Make a longitudinal incision over the area of greatest fluctuance (either on the volar aspect or laterally) into the pulp space of the fingertip. Do not extend the incision proximal to the mid-portion of the distal phalanx in order to avoid injury to the flexor tendon or the joint space. Care should also be taken to avoid injury to the digital arteries and nerves, which run together in a neurovascular bundle (Fig. 44–2*B*).
4. Allow purulent fluid to drain from the wound, and place either a small portion of a Penrose drain or packing material to act as a wick to allow for continued drainage (Fig. 44–2*C*).
5. The lateral incision can be extended to the tip of the finger ("hockey stick incision") or through the pulp space to the other side of the digit for especially well-developed infections (Fig. 44–3).
6. Bandage the finger with an absorbent dressing.
7. Follow-up should occur in 24 to 48 hr, at which time the drain or wick can be removed and the patient can begin daily warm water soaks. The incision is allowed to heal by secondary intention.

COMPLICATIONS

1. Injury to the flexor tendon mechanism or distal interphalangeal (DIP) joint space
2. Injury to the neurovascular bundle (distal digital nerve and artery)
3. Bacteremia and septicemia
4. Increasing cellulitis following the procedure
5. Bleeding

References

Hausman MR, Lisser SP. Hand infections. Orthop Clin North Am 23(1):171–185, 1992.
Roberts JR, Hedges JR. *Clinical Procedures in Emergency Medicine* (2nd ed). Philadelphia, WB Saunders, 1991, pp 605–608.
Trott A. *Wounds and Lacerations: Emergency Care and Closure.* St. Louis, Mosby-Year Book, 1991, pp 210–211.

CHAPTER 45

Steven Krug

NAIL TREPHINATION— DRAINAGE OF SUBUNGUAL HEMATOMA

INDICATIONS

1. Pain relief from and drainage of subungual hematoma

CONTRAINDICATIONS

1. Severely injured or lacerated nailbed

NOTE: While subungual hematomas are frequently associated with a laceration of the nailbed, examination of the nailbed (i.e., lifting the nail), and repair of a nailbed laceration is not indicated for "uncomplicated" hematomas.

EQUIPMENT

1. Battery powered heat cautery device (alternatively, one can use a heated paper clip)
2. Scalpel, #11 blade
3. Povidone-iodine solution
4. Gloves

PROCEDURE

1. Although this procedure can typically be completed without anesthesia, consider providing a digital nerve block (see Chapter 40, on regional nerve blocks).
2. Consider obtaining a radiograph to establish the presence of a fracture.

NOTE: The presence of a distal phalanx fracture and a nailbed laceration or

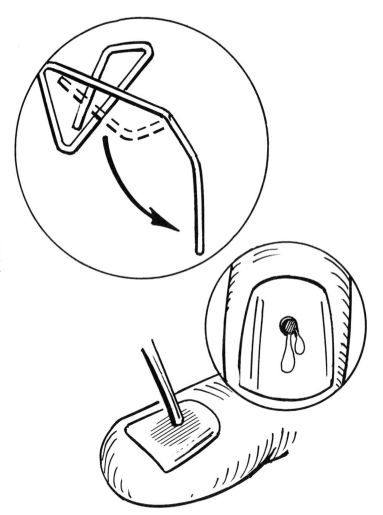

Figure 45–1. Drainage of subungual hematoma can be accomplished either by a portable cautery device or by the use of a heated paper clip.

Figure 45–2. Hematoma may also be drained using a #11 scalpel blade.

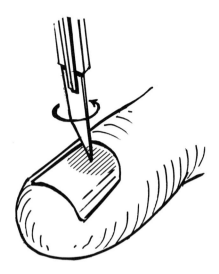

subungual hematoma is by definition an open fracture. The benefits of antibiotic prophylaxis have not been established for this situation.

3. Consider lifting the nail to examine for significant nailbed injuries.
4. Clean the surface of the nail with povidone-iodine solution.
5. Make one or more holes in the nail using a portable heat cautery device or a heated paperclip. If a single puncture is made, take care to make a hole large enough to allow for continued drainage (Fig. 45-1).
6. An alternative to the technique using a heated paperclip or cautery device is a #11 scalpel blade. The tip of the blade is placed on the nail and a small hole is created by applying both downward pressure and a rotary motion of the blade (Fig. 45-2).

COMPLICATIONS

1. Osteomyelitis (due to an open fracture)
2. Bleeding

References

Ruddy RM (ed). Illustrated techniques of pediatric emergency procedures. In Fleisher GR, Ludwig S (eds): *Textbook of Pediatric Emergency Medicine* (3rd ed). Baltimore, Williams & Wilkins, 1993.
Warden TM, Fourré MW. Incision and drainage of cutaneous abscesses and soft tissue infections. In Roberts JR, Hedges JR (eds). *Clinical Procedures in Emergency Medicine* (2nd ed). Philadelphia, WB Saunders, 1991.

CHAPTER 46

Steven Krug

REMOVAL OF A SUBUNGUAL FOREIGN BODY—SPLINTER

INDICATIONS

1. Removal of (and pain relief from) a subungual foreign body

CONTRAINDICATIONS

None

EQUIPMENT

1. Scalpel #11 blade
2. Fine forceps
3. Povidone-iodine solution
4. Syringe, 3- to 5-cc
5. 25- or 27-gauge needle, 1 to 2 in
6. 1% lidocaine (without epinephrine)
7. 8.4% sodium bicarbonate—may be mixed with the lidocaine in a 1:9 parts ratio (1 part $NaHCO_3$ to 9 parts lidocaine) to reduce the pain associated with injection
8. Gloves

PROCEDURE

1. Provide analgesia for the procedure using a digital block. Ensure sufficient restraint of the patient.
2. Clean the surface of the nail with povidone-iodine solution.
3. Using the scalpel blade, scrape the area of the nail that lies over the foreign object down to the nailbed (Fig. 46–1). The goal is to remove a small wedge of nail over the splinter.
4. Remove the splinter with fine forceps (Fig. 46–2).

NOTE: For certain splinter materials, one may only need to scrape down the nail

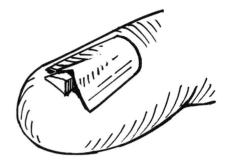

Figure 46–1. A small wedge of nail overlying the splinter should be removed with the scalpel.

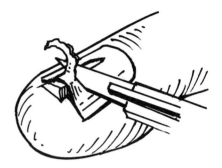

overlying the distal aspect of the splinter, thereby allowing access with forceps to pull out the splinter.

COMPLICATIONS

1. Infection
2. Hemorrhage

References

Lammers RL. Principles of wound management. In Roberts JR, Hedges JR (eds). *Clinical Procedures in Emergency Medicine* (2nd ed). Philadelphia, WB Saunders, 1991.
Ruddy RM (ed). Illustrated techniques of pediatric emergency procedures. In Fleisher GR, Ludwig S (eds). *Textbook of Pediatric Emergency Medicine* (3rd ed). Baltimore, Williams & Wilkins, 1993.

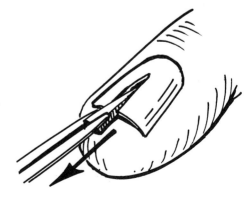

Figure 46–2. Foreign body is removed with fine forceps.

Steven Krug

CHAPTER 47

FISHHOOK REMOVAL

INDICATIONS

1. Removal of fishhook embedded in the skin

CONTRAINDICATIONS

None

EQUIPMENT

1. Povidone-iodine solution
2. 1% lidocaine (preferably buffered)
3. 5-cc syringe with 25- or 27-gauge needle
4. Needle holders
5. Gloves

PROCEDURES

Cutting of Hook Barb

1. This procedure is ideal for small hooks that are located fairly superficially.
2. After preparing the skin, the skin overlying the barb and the area where the barb is anticipated to be pushed through the skin should be infiltrated with lidocaine (Fig. 47–1*A*).
3. Upon completion of local anesthesia, the point of the hook should be forced through the skin (Fig. 47–1*B*).
4. The barb should then be cut with a wirecutter (Fig. 47–1*C*).
5. The remainder of the hook can then be removed by reversing the direction of entry (Fig. 47–1*D*).

Needle Sheathing of Hook Barb

1. For larger or deeper hooks, this method may be preferred over the barb cut.
2. After preparing the skin, provide adequate local anesthesia at the site of skin entry (Fig. 47–2*A*).

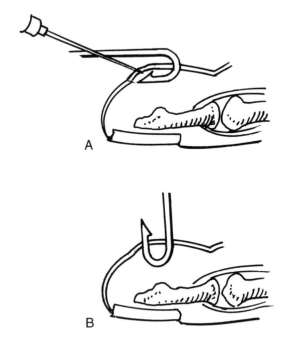

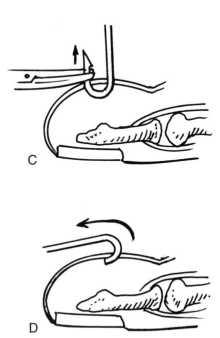

Figure 47–1. Cutting off the hook barb. This technique is ideal for smaller or superficially located hooks.

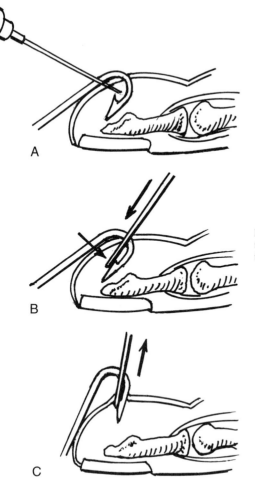

Figure 47–2. The needle sheathing technique may be preferred for larger or deeply embedded hooks. See text for details.

3. Using an 18-gauge needle, pass the needle with the bevel down through the hook's entry wound. Keep the needle parallel to the shank of the hook until it reaches the barb (Fig. 47-2*B*).
4. With the barb covered, the hook may now be removed in tandem with the needle (Fig. 47-2*C*).

String ("Fishing Stream") Method

1. As the name suggests, this technique can be accomplished with no local anesthesia, although it is generally prudent to provide local infiltration of 1% lidocaine at the entry site.
2. Loop a segment of string or heavy suture around the hook.
3. One or two fingers from the nondominant hand should be used to press the shaft of the hook against the skin (Fig. 47-3*A*). This helps to disengage the barb.
4. Grasping the string with the dominant hand, pull sharply in a direction opposite to the route of entry (Fig. 47-3*B*). The hook should exit the skin at its entry site. As this procedure may result in a very rapid and poorly controlled exit of the hook, great care should be taken to avoid this hazardous projectile.

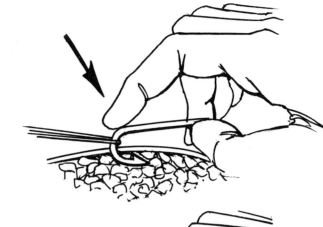

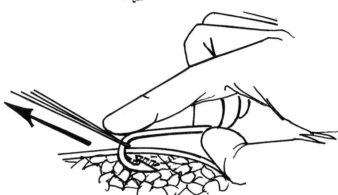

Figure 47–3. "Fishing stream" method for fishhook removal.

COMPLICATIONS

1. Trauma to skin and underlying structures
2. Infection
3. Hemorrhage

References

Barnett RC. Soft tissue foreign body removal. In Roberts JR, Hedges JR (eds). *Clinical Procedures in Emergency Medicine* (2nd ed). Philadelphia, WB Saunders, 1991.
Ruddy RM (ed). Illustrated techniques of pediatric emergency procedures. In Fleisher GR, Ludwig S (eds). *Textbook of Pediatric Emergency Medicine* (3rd ed). Baltimore, Williams & Wilkins, 1993.

CHAPTER 48

Steven Krug

RING REMOVAL

INDICATIONS

1. Presence of a strangulating ring on a digit

CONTRAINDICATIONS

None

EQUIPMENT

1. Ring cutter
2. Suture
3. Lubricant

PROCEDURES

Ring Cutting

1. Place the ring cutter guard between the ring and the finger. Close the ring cutter, placing the blade on the ring.
2. Applying pressure to the handle of the ring cutter, turn the blade until the ring has been cut (Fig. 48-1).
3. The ring may then be removed by pulling it apart manually with the assistance of a hemostat. Occasionally, the ring will need to be cut a second time to allow this.
4. Patients with significant pain or edema may require a digital block or conscious sedation.

String Finger Compression

1. Consider placing a digital block or providing conscious sedation and analgesia.
2. If possible, move the ring to the most proximal aspect of the segment of the digit it is stuck on (e.g., to the proximal interphalangeal or metacarpophalangeal joint).
3. Using fine string or 3-0 suture, wrap the string around the finger, starting at the fingertip. Wrap the string tightly and continue winding in a proximal direction until the ring is reached.
4. Grasp the ring and pull or twist it over the suture and then off of the finger (Fig. 48-2). If the ring fails to pull completely off the finger, pull the string around and off the finger at the proximal end. This will pull the ring off the finger.

Suture Pull

1. Consider placing a digital block or providing conscious sedation and analgesia.
2. Using a heavy suture grade (1-0 silk or better), run one end of the suture between the ring and the finger. Loop the ends of the suture together.
3. Place a generous amount of lubricant on the finger distal to the ring.
4. Using a continuous circular motion, pull the suture around the finger. This should cause the ring to gradually slip off the finger (Fig. 48-3).

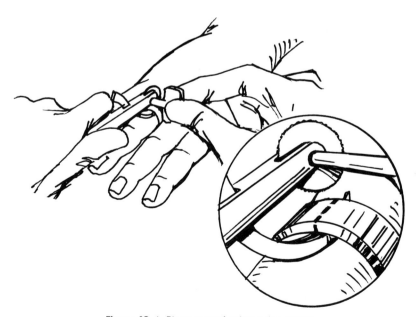

Figure 48–1. Ring removal using a ring cutter.

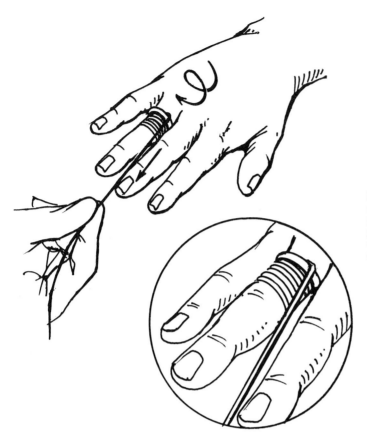

Figure 48–2. Whenever possible, move ring to most proximal aspect of the digit prior to wrapping suture around the finger. The use of a digital block and a generous amount of lubricant will assist a successful outcome.

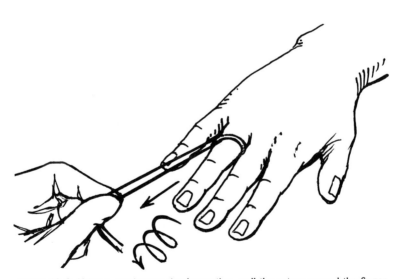

Figure 48–3. Using a continuous circular motion, pull the suture around the finger.

COMPLICATIONS

1. Trauma to the digit
2. Neurovascular compromise

References

Barnett RC. Soft tissue foreign body removal. In Roberts JR, Hedges JR (eds). *Clinical Procedures in Emergency Medicine* (2nd ed). Philadelphia, WB Saunders, 1991.
Ruddy RM (ed). Illustrated techniques of pediatric emergency procedures. In Fleisher GR, Ludwig S (eds). *Textbook of Pediatric Emergency Medicine* (3rd ed). Baltimore, Williams & Wilkins, 1993.

CHAPTER 49

Ian McCaslin

TREATMENT OF MINOR BURNS

INDICATIONS

Burn severity is characterized by the depth of the burn and by the percentage of body surface area (BSA) involved. Degree of burn injury is an evolving process and often cannot be determined absolutely at the time of presentation. First-degree burns involve the epidermis only and are usually not blistered initially, whereas second-degree burns extend into the dermis. Partial thickness second-degree burns are blistered, pink, moist, and painful, whereas deep second-degree burns are often white, dry, and nonblanching. Third-degree burns extend into the subcutaneous tissues; have a white, leathery, or charred appearance; and are typically painless. Children over 2 years old with partial-thickness second-degree burns of less than 10% BSA can generally be managed as outpatients, whether by primary care or by emergency physicians, provided the family is compliant with dressing changes and follow-up.

CONTRAINDICATIONS

Some injuries or circumstances should generally be managed in the hospital. These would include:

1. Burns of certain anatomic areas; for example, perineum, hands, feet, or face
2. Suspected abuse
3. Deep burn greater than 3% BSA
4. Circumferential burns
5. Burns that cross a joint line
6. Uncertain follow-up

Transfer to a specialized burn center is indicated for:

1. Burns of greater than 20% BSA
2. When intensive care monitoring is anticipated, as with inhalation injury or high-voltage electrical burn

EQUIPMENT

1. Sterile gloves
2. Mild soap or Hibiclens

3. Saline solution
4. Forceps and scissors
5. Sterile tongue depressor
6. Antibiotic ointment (e.g., Silvadene, Bacitracin, or Neosporin)
7. Nonadherent porous dressing such as Adaptic, Aquaphor, Telfa, or Xeroform
8. Kerlix wrapping
9. Paper tape

PROCEDURE

1. Scene management includes initial cooling in room temperature water, followed by wrapping in a soaked clean sheet or moistened gauze pads.
2. In the emergency department, ensure adequate pain relief.
3. Cleanse the burned area with mild soap and cool water or with Hibiclens diluted with saline.
4. Hair should not be shaved from the area. Debride obviously sloughed skin and open blisters, preferably with a quick swipe of a dry gauze pad. Leave intact blisters alone, unless infection is obvious.
5. Apply a thin layer of topical antibiotic ointment with a sterile tongue depressor and cover with a nonadherent porous dressing material. An alternate approach is to cover the burn directly with Xeroform. Neither biologic nor synthetic dressings are routinely required for minor burns in children.
6. Protect the dressing with bulky gauze pads and wrap with Kerlix secured by paper tape.
7. Provide tetanus prophylaxis if indicated.
8. Neither steroids nor prophylactic antibiotics are initially indicated.
9. Teach caretakers to change dressing one to two times daily. Provide the materials and written instructions for dressing changes.
10. Emphasize follow-up in 48 hr with a physician.

COMPLICATIONS

1. Infection
2. Joint contracture
3. Underrecognition of full-thickness burn requiring skin grafting
4. Scarring
5. Functional impairment

References

Baxter CR, Waeckerle JF. Emergency treatment of burn injury. Ann Emerg Med 17:1305-1315, 1988.
Schonfeld N. Outpatient management of burns in children. Pediatr Emerg Care 6:249-253, 1990.
Warden GD. Outpatient management of thermal injuries. In Boswick JA (ed). *The Art and Science of Burn Care*. Rockville, MD, Aspen Publishers, 1987.

SECTION 6

ORTHOPEDICS

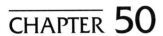

CHAPTER **50**

Steven Krug

SPLINTING OF MUSCULOSKELETAL INJURIES—PLASTER SPLINTS

INDICATIONS

1. Short-term immobilization, stabilization, and protection of musculoskeletal injuries such as sprains, strains, fractures, dislocations, and lacerations
2. Location and splint specific
   a. Thumb spica—simple fractures (nonangulated, nonrotated, and nonarticular) of the first metacarpal or phalanx, gamekeeper's thumb (ulnar collateral ligament injury), scaphoid fracture
   b. Ulnar gutter—simple boxer's fracture (<20 degrees angulation), simple fractures of the fourth or fifth phalanges.
   c. Forearm sugar-tong splint—simple fractures of the distal radius and/or ulna
   d. Long arm posterior—elbow and forearm injuries
   e. Ankle posterior—ankle sprains and fractures of the foot, ankle, and distal fibula
   f. Long leg posterior—knee injuries and fractures of the tibia and fibula

CONTRAINDICATIONS

1. Open and complex (angulated, rotated, articular) fractures—These all require orthopedic evaluation.
2. Evidence of impaired distal neurovascular function

EQUIPMENT

1. Cotton bandage (Webril)
2. Stockinette
3. Plaster—may be in precut slabs or in rolls—2- through 6-in widths; pre-padded plaster splinting material (OCL) is an option
4. Water bucket
5. Elastic bandages
7. Adhesive tape
8. Slings (for upper-extremity injuries)
9. Crutches—for age-appropriate lower-extremity injuries

PROCEDURES

General Considerations

1. Confirm the presence of normal neurovascular function of the affected extremity, both proximal and distal to the injury. Abnormal function warrants orthopedic consultation.
2. Determine the style and length of splint required. Generally a splint should provide for immobilization of one joint proximal and one joint distal to the injury. Use a tape measure to accurately determine the actual length of plaster needed.
3. Become familiar with anatomic position of function. Extremities must be splinted in such a manner as to minimize contractures.
4. Clean, repair, and dress all skin wounds in the area to be splinted prior to putting on the splint. If an open fracture is suspected, obtain orthopedic consultation.
5. Choose a width of plaster that allows for coverage of approximately half the circumference of the affected extremity.

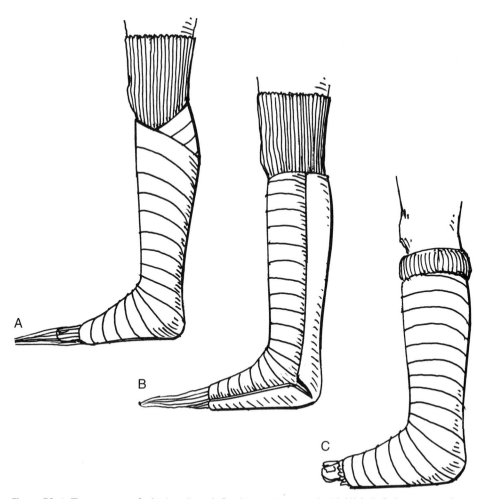

Figure 50–1. The anatomy of a basic splint. *A*, Stockinette is covered with Webril. *B*, A posterior plaster mold maintains limb in neutral position. *C*, Ace wrap secures splint in place. Take care not to wrap the bandage too tightly.

6. If you are using plaster rolls or slabs, upper extremities will require 8 to 10 layers of plaster, whereas the lower extremities warrant 12 to 14 layers.
7. Once the plaster has been cut, prepare the padding for the splint. A Webril bandage should be rolled around the portion of the extremity to be splinted in a distal-to-proximal direction. The rolls should allow for an overlap of approximately 50%. This padding should extend well beyond the splinted area (2 to 3 cm) (Fig. 50-1A). Special attention should be paid to bony prominences, which may require additional padding. If digits are to be included in the splinted area, padding should be placed between digits.

NOTE: As an option, stockinette dressing may be placed on the area of the limb to be splinted before the application of Webril.

8. The plaster should be immersed in room temperature water until the bubbling stops (approximately 15 to 20 sec). Then remove the plaster and smooth it out on a flat surface so as to remove excess water and wrinkles and to bond the plaster layers.
9. Apply the splint to the extremity, molding it into a position of function. Mold the splint to the contours of the extremity, taking care not to create indentations (Fig. 50-1B).
10. Fold the exposed Webril (and stockinette if present) at each end of the splint over and onto the borders of the splint.
11. Roll an elastic bandage over the splint in a distal to proximal direction. Take care not to wrap the bandage too tightly (Fig. 50-1C).
12. Note that applying the Ace wrap directly to the plaster may result in its sticking to the plaster. To prevent this, consider placing a layer of Webril between the plaster and the elastic bandage. This may be accomplished using a circumferential roll technique or by layering Webril over the plaster itself.

Thumb Spica

1. Splint will extend along the radial aspect of the forearm from the thumbnail to 3 to 4 cm distal to the volar crease of the elbow. The U-shaped splint must be wide enough to completely encircle the thumb (Fig. 50-2).
2. Position of function should maintain the wrist in slight dorsiflexion, with the thumb in abduction, and the first interphalangeal joint in slight flexion. The splint should be applied with the elbow in a neutral position (i.e., no pronation or supination).

Ulnar Gutter

1. Splint will extend along the ulnar aspect of the forearm from the distal interphalangeal joint to 3 to 4 cm distal to the volar crease of the elbow. The U-shaped splint must be wide enough to completely encircle the fourth and fifth digits and overlie both the volar and dorsal surfaces of the fourth and fifth metacarpals (Fig. 50-3).
2. Position of function should maintain the wrist in slight dorsiflexion, 50 to 90 degrees flexion of the fourth and fifth digits at the metacarpophalangeal joint, and 20 degrees of flexion at the interphalangeal joints. The splint should be applied with the elbow in a neutral position (no pronation or supination).

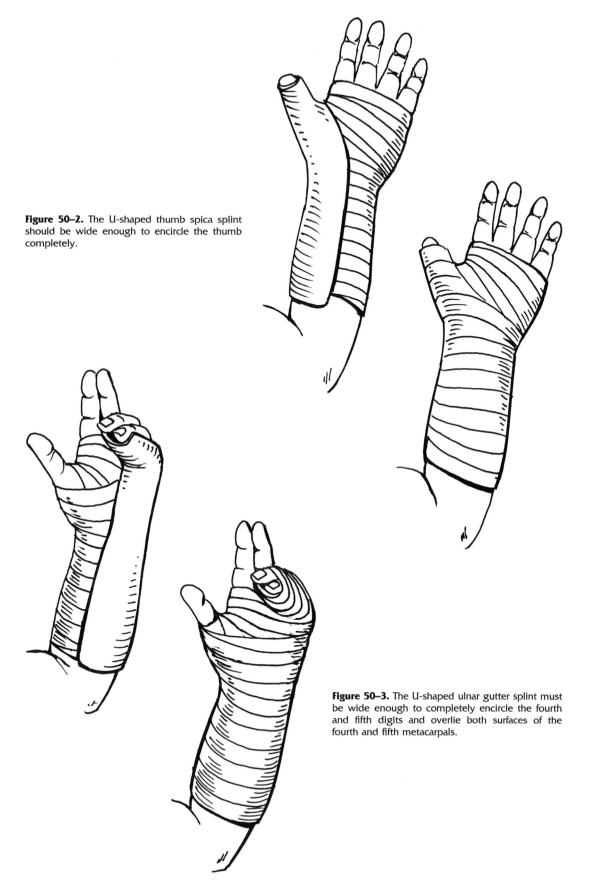

Figure 50–2. The U-shaped thumb spica splint should be wide enough to encircle the thumb completely.

Figure 50–3. The U-shaped ulnar gutter splint must be wide enough to completely encircle the fourth and fifth digits and overlie both surfaces of the fourth and fifth metacarpals.

Forearm Sugartong

1. Splint will extend from the volar aspect of the metacarpophalangeal joints around the elbow to the dorsal surface of the metacarpophalangeal joints (Fig. 50-4).
2. Position of function should maintain the wrist in slight dorsiflexion and the forearm flexed at 90 degrees at the elbow in a neutral position (no pronation or supination). The fingers should be free to have full range of motion.

Long Arm Posterior

1. Splint will extend from the level of the mid-metacarpal over the ulnar aspect of the forearm and elbow to approximately one third the distance up the upper arm from the elbow (Fig. 50-5). The splint should be wide enough to cover about half the circumference of the arm.
2. Position of function should maintain the elbow at 90 degrees of flexion in a neutral position (no pronation or supination).

Ankle Posterior

1. Splint will extend from the level of the metatarsophalangeal joint on the volar aspect of the foot behind the ankle up to 3 to 4 cm below the knee (Fig. 50-6).
2. Position of function maintains the ankle in 90 degrees of flexion and the foot and toes in a neutral position.

Long Leg Posterior

1. Splint will extend from the level of the metatarsophalangeal joint on the volar aspect of the foot behind the ankle and knee up to 3 to 4 cm before the gluteal fold (Fig. 50-7).
2. Position of function maintains the ankle in 90 degrees of flexion and the knee, foot, and toes in a neutral position.

COMPLICATIONS

1. Neurovascular compromise
2. Reduction of joint function (caused by prolonged immobilization) or contractures
3. Contact or pressure-induced skin ulcers
4. Contact dermatitis
5. Reinjury due to inadequate immobilization

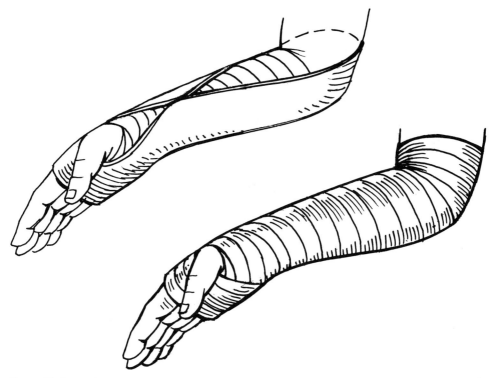

Figure 50–4. The forearm sugar tong is an effective means to immobilize simple fractures of the distal radius and/or ulna.

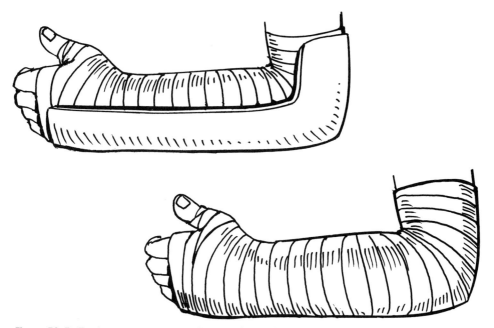

Figure 50–5. The long arm posterior splint may be used to immobilize proximal forearm and elbow injuries.

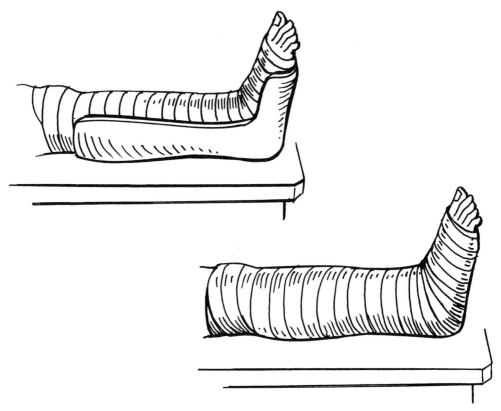

Figure 50–6. The posterior ankle splint may be used to immobilize ankle sprains and fractures of the foot, ankle, and distal fibula.

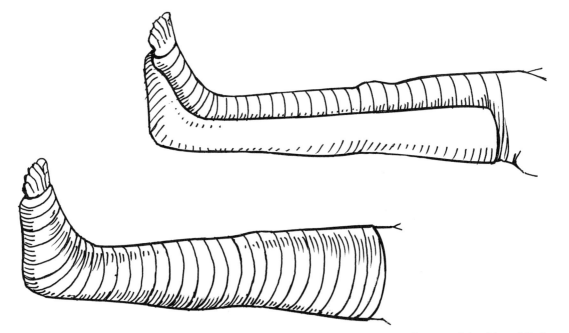

Figure 50–7. The long leg posterior splint may be used to immobilize knee injuries and fractures of the tibia and fibula.

References

Chudnofsky CR, Otten EJ, Newmeyer WL. Splinting techniques. In Roberts JR, Hedges JR (eds). *Clinical Procedures in Emergency Medicine* (2nd ed). Philadelphia, WB Saunders, 1991.

Ruddy RM (ed). Illustrated techniques of pediatric emergency procedures. In Fleisher GR, Ludwig S (eds). *Textbook of Pediatric Emergency Medicine* (3rd ed). Baltimore, Williams & Wilkins, 1993.

Simon RR, Koenigsknecht SJ. *Emergency Orthopedics—The Extremities* (3rd ed). Norwalk, CT, Appleton and Lange, 1995.

Steven Krug

SPLINTING OF MUSCULOSKELETAL INJURIES—FINGER SPLINTS

INDICATIONS

1. Immobilization of the phalanx for simple fractures, lacerations, or sprains of the interphalangeal joints

CONTRAINDICATIONS

1. Finger injuries requiring orthopedic evaluation
   a. Fractures resulting in rotary or angulated deformities
   b. Fractures involving greater than 10% of an articular surface
   c. Mallet, gamekeeper's, or boutonnière injuries

EQUIPMENT

1. Aluminum splints with foam padding, varied widths
2. Adhesive tape, ½- and 1-in widths

PROCEDURES

Dorsal Splint

1. Splint should extend from the dorsum of the wrist at the level of the carpal-metacarpal joint to the end of the injured finger. Note that dorsal splints are preferred over volar splints as they serve to maintain tactile sensation (Fig. 51–1).
2. Measure and cut the necessary length of splint. Cover exposed sharp edges with 1-in tape.
3. Position of comfort should maintain the metacarpophalangeal joint in 50 to 90 degrees of flexion and the interphalangeal joints in 15 to 20 degrees of flexion.
4. Attach the splint using ½-in tape. Do not place tape over joint lines or over the distal phalanx.

Dynamic Splint

1. This technique provides immobilization of phalangeal injuries while allowing for motion at the metacarpophalangeal joint.

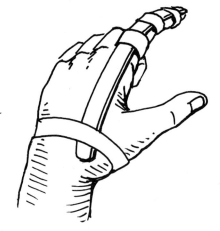

Figure 51–1. The dorsal splint should extend from the level of the carpo-metacarpal joint to the end of the injured finger.

2. The injured finger is splinted to an adjacent noninjured finger using ½- to 1-inch tape (Fig. 51–2). A piece of felt or foam may be placed between the two fingers before taping.

COMPLICATIONS

1. Neurovascular compromise
2. Reduction of joint function (owing to prolonged immobilization) or contractures
3. Contact or pressure-induced skin ulcers
4. Contact dermatitis
5. Reinjury due to inadequate immobilization

References

Chudnofsky CR, Otten EJ, Newmeyer WL. Splinting techniques. In Roberts JR, Hedges JR (eds). *Clinical Procedures in Emergency Medicine* (2nd ed). Philadelphia, WB Saunders, 1991.

Ruddy RM (ed). Illustrated techniques of pediatric emergency procedures. In Fleisher GR, Ludwig S (eds). *Textbook of Pediatric Emergency Medicine* (3rd ed). Baltimore, Williams & Wilkins, 1993.

Simon RR, Koenigsknecht SJ. *Emergency Orthopedics—The Extremities* (3rd ed). Norwalk, CT, Appleton and Lange, 1995.

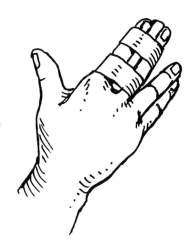

Figure 51–2. The dynamic splint technique provides immobilization while allowing for motion at the metacarpophalangeal joint.

SPLINTING OF MUSCULOSKELETAL INJURIES—FIGURE-OF-EIGHT HARNESS

INDICATIONS

1. Immobilization of a midshaft fracture of the clavicle. Note that the primary benefit to the patient is that of comfort, as these injuries will heal well without splinting.

CONTRAINDICATIONS

1. Fractures of the medial or distal third of the clavicle (sling is the preferred method for distal third injuries)

EQUIPMENT

1. Commercially available figure-of-eight harness, various sizes

PROCEDURES

1. Confirm presence and location of clavicle fracture.
2. Choose appropriate-sized harness device.
3. With the child standing and facing away, drape the harness over the shoulders. Manually adjust the straps to provide for a symmetric shortening of the straps. The harness should fit snugly (Fig. 52–1).
4. The proper position is one in which the shoulders are straight and are pulled back from their usual forward, rounded position.

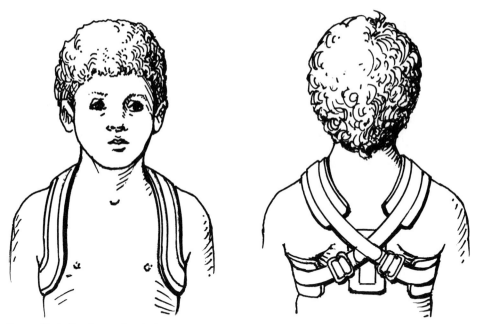

Figure 52–1. The figure-of-eight harness may provide for comfort for the child with a clavicle fracture. If the harness is unavailable, a sling may be used in its place.

COMPLICATIONS

1. Pressure sore
2. Pain (incorrect or loose application)

References

Ruddy RM (ed). Illustrated techniques of pediatric emergency procedures. In Fleisher GR, Ludwig S (eds). *Textbook of Pediatric Emergency Medicine* (3rd ed). Baltimore, Williams & Wilkins, 1993.
Simon RR, Koenigsknecht SJ. *Emergency Orthopedics—The Extremities* (3rd ed). Norwalk, CT, Appleton and Lange, 1995.

Steven Krug

SPLINTING OF MUSCULOSKELETAL INJURIES—SLINGS

INDICATIONS

1. Elevation and immobilization of the hand, forearm, elbow, upper arm, shoulder
2. Support of arm for a variety of injuries in conjunction with a splint or cast
3. Distal third clavicle fractures
4. Fracture of the proximal humerus (sling and swath)

CONTRAINDICATIONS

1. None

EQUIPMENT

1. Commercial sling
2. Triangular bandage, stockinette, and wide elastic bandage
3. Velpeau bandage (sling and swath)

PROCEDURES

Simple Sling

1. A simple sling may be created from a triangular bandage (or a commercial sling) which is folded in half and tied around the neck.
2. The sling should be large or wide enough so that it provides support for the forearm, wrist, and hand.
3. For typical use to support casted or splinted injuries, the sling should be adjusted so that it maintains the forearm in a horizontal position (Fig. 53–1).
4. If the sling is to be used to promote elevation of a hand or forearm injury, the sling should be shortened to position the forearm diagonally at a 30- to 45-degree angle to the horizontal plane.

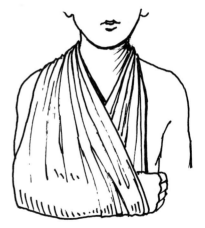

Figure 53–1. The sling should be wide enough so that it provides support for the entire forearm, wrist, and hand.

Sling and Swath (Velpeau Bandage)

1. The Velpeau bandage is applied much like a standard sling, with the exception that the forearm is supported in a position that is diagonal to a horizontal plane. Optimally, the hand should be elevated to the level of the shoulder (Fig. 53-2).
2. The swath or an elastic bandage is then used to secure the sling to the patient's torso. The swath should wrap snugly and encircle the patient's torso and the immobilized extremity.

COMPLICATIONS

1. Swelling or pain secondary to improper immobilization (e.g., a sling that allows the hand to dangle) or inadequate elevation.

References

Chudnofsky CR, Otten EJ, Newmeyer WL. Splinting techniques. In Roberts JR, Hedges JR (eds). *Clinical Procedures in Emergency Medicine* (2nd ed). Philadelphia, WB Saunders, 1991.

Ruddy RM (ed). Illustrated techniques of pediatric emergency procedures. In Fleisher GR, Ludwig S (eds). *Textbook of Pediatric Emergency Medicine* (3rd ed). Baltimore, Williams & Wilkins, 1993.

Simon RR, Koenigsknecht SJ. *Emergency Orthopedics—The Extremities* (3rd ed). Norwalk, CT, Appleton and Lange, 1995.

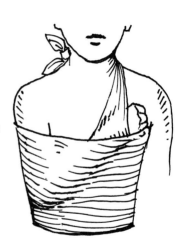

Figure 53–2. The sling and swath are used as a method of choice to immobilize proximal humerus fractures.

CHAPTER 54

Cynthia Hoecker

REDUCTION OF RADIAL HEAD SUBLUXATION ("NURSEMAID'S ELBOW")

INDICATIONS

Radial head subluxation is a condition occurring in infants and toddlers that results from axial traction on the arm, causing the radial head to be displaced from under the annular ligament (Fig. 54-1). Usually there is a history of extension of the arm followed by refusal to use the arm, which the child holds at his or her side in a slightly flexed and pronated position. There is no swelling or bruising of the arm with this condition. An attempt at manual reduction is recommended in children who present with a such a history and an absence of external signs of trauma.

CONTRAINDICATIONS

1. External signs of trauma to the upper extremity (swelling, ecchymosis)
2. Suspicion or confirmation of elbow or forearm fracture/dislocation
3. Known mechanism of injury unlikely to result in radial head subluxation

EQUIPMENT

None

PROCEDURE

1. The examiner's thumb is placed over the radial head as the rest of the hand rests on the underside of the proximal forearm (Fig. 54-2).
2. The examiner's other hand is used to supinate the child's hand while applying axial traction at the wrist and beginning to flex the child's arm at the elbow (Fig. 54-3).
3. Firm pressure is placed by the examiner's thumb over the radial head as the arm is being flexed and the supinated hand is raised toward the shoulder (Fig. 54-4).
4. Usually a click is felt near the elbow as the radial head pops back under the ligament.

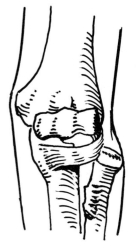

Figure 54–1. Axial traction on the hand or forearm of a preschool-aged child with the elbow in an extended position can result in subluxation of the radial head.

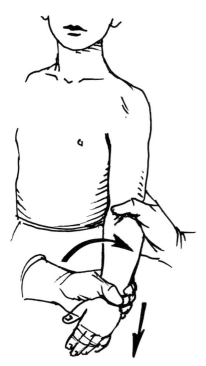

Figure 54–2. Reduction of the radial head subluxation begins with axial traction applied to the forearm with the wrist adducted to the ulnar side. Pressure is also applied directly over the radial head at the level of the antecubital fossa.

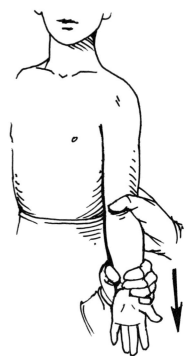

Figure 54–3. The forearm is supinated while axial traction and pressure are maintained over the radial head.

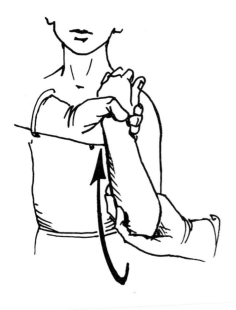

Figure 54–4. The forearm is then flexed while supination and pressure are maintained over the radial head.

5. The child is observed for approximately 15 to 20 min, during which time he or she should regain use of the arm.
6. If the child's use of the arm is not improved, either a second attempt at reduction may be undertaken or an x-ray examination may be obtained before further attempts at manual reduction, in order to rule out an orthopedic injury.

COMPLICATIONS

Neurovascular injury resulting from manipulation of the arm when there is a fracture or dislocation

References

Michaels MG. A case of bilateral nursemaid's elbow. Pediatr Emerg Care 5(4):226–227, 1989.
Sachetti A, et al. Non-classic history in children with radial head subluxations. J Emerg Med 8:151–153, 1990.
Schunk JE. Radial head subluxation: Epidemiology and treatment of 87 episodes. Ann Emerg Med 19(9):10, 19–1023, 1990.
Snyder HS. Radiographic changes with radial head subluxation in children. J Emerg Med 8:265–269, 1990.

CHAPTER 55

Steven Krug

DISLOCATION REDUCTION—ANTERIOR SHOULDER

INDICATIONS

1. Anterior dislocation of the humeral head (Fig. 55-1)
   a. Subcoracoid (most common type)
   b. Subglenoid
   c. Subclavicular
2. Typical findings in patients with an anterior dislocation include the arm held to the side, with loss of the normal rounded contour of the shoulder. The patient will resist any effort at internal rotation and adduction.

CONTRAINDICATIONS

1. Presence of associated fracture to the humeral head or glenoid fossa; these warrant urgent orthopedic consultation
2. Patients with significant neurovascular compromise of the affected extremity; these too warrant orthopedic consultation

EQUIPMENT

1. Bedsheets
2. Counterweight
3. Sling and swath

PROCEDURES

Hennepin or External Rotation Method

NOTE: In cooperative patients, many authors think that this is the procedure of choice for the reduction of anterior shoulder dislocations. The technique allows the shoulder muscles to essentially "self-reduce" the dislocation and requires little manipulation and brute force on the physician's part.

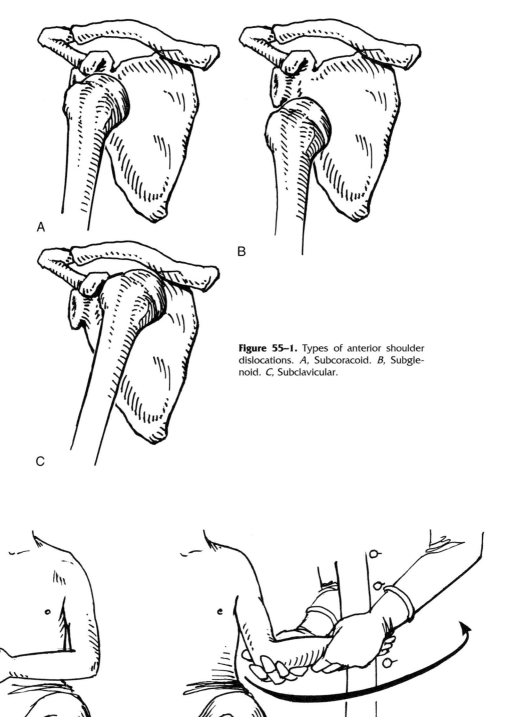

Figure 55–1. Types of anterior shoulder dislocations. *A*, Subcoracoid. *B*, Subglenoid. *C*, Subclavicular.

Figure 55–2. The Hennepin or external rotation method is the technique of choice for reduction of anterior shoulder dislocation in a cooperative patient.

1. Confirm the diagnosis of anterior shoulder dislocation and the absence of an associated fracture with radiographs. Consider the use of sedation and analgesia.
2. This procedure can occur with the patient either in a sitting or supine position.
3. With the affected arm adducted to the patient's side, the elbow of the affected extremity is flexed to 90 degrees with the forearm in a sagittal plane (Fig. 55-2A).
4. Using the forearm as a lever, the arm is slowly externally rotated (Fig. 55-2B). If pain is experienced, rotation should be halted until the shoulder muscles relax and the pain remits.
5. The arm is rotated until it reaches 90 degrees. Reduction is usually achieved once the coronal plane has been reached.
6. If reduction has not occurred, the arm may be elevated until the humeral head re-enters the joint.
7. Post reduction care should include radiographs, reassessment of neurovascular function, and the application of a sling and swath.

Stimson Maneuver

NOTE: In cooperative patients, this is an excellent procedure, as it allows the force of gravity to gradually overcome the muscle spasm associated with an anterior shoulder dislocation and does so with a very small risk of injury to the patient, and typically without excessive analgesia.

1. Confirm the diagnosis of anterior shoulder dislocation, and the absence of an associated fracture with radiographs. Consider the use of sedation and analgesia.
2. The patient is placed in a prone position on a gurney, with the arm of the dislocated shoulder hanging over the edge of the bed.
3. A 10- to 20-lb weight is attached to the wrist or arm in a fashion to allow it to provide constant traction (Fig. 55-3). This weight is left undisturbed for 20 to 30 min, or until the shoulder has been reduced.
4. If this procedure fails to reduce the joint, gentle external and internal rotation of the shoulder joint during the traction may assist reduction.
5. Post reduction care should include radiographs, reassessment of neurovascular function, and the application of a sling and swath.

Traction–Countertraction

1. Confirm the diagnosis of anterior shoulder dislocation, and the absence of an associated fracture with radiographs. Consider sedation and analgesia.
2. The patient is placed in a supine position on a gurney.
3. Countertraction is provided by a bedsheet that is wrapped around the patient's upper chest and under the axilla of the affected shoulder (Fig. 55-4). This sheet is either tied to the bed or held by an assistant.
4. A second sheet or strap is placed around the flexed forearm of the affected extremity, just distal to the elbow.
5. Gentle in-line traction on this sheet (which can be tied around the waist of the physician, who then leans back away from the patient, providing traction) should slowly counteract muscle spasm and result in reduction of the humeral head.
6. A related method employs direct axial traction on the extended extremity, rather than using the sheet tied around the forearm (Fig. 55-5).

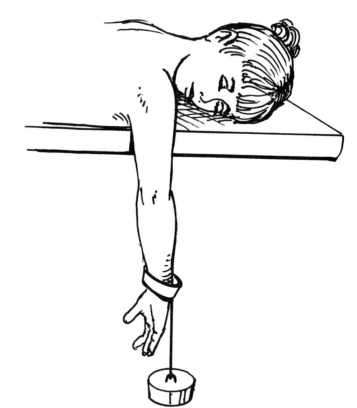

Figure 55–3. Stimson method for reduction of anterior shoulder dislocation. This technique may be successful without excessive sedation or analgesia.

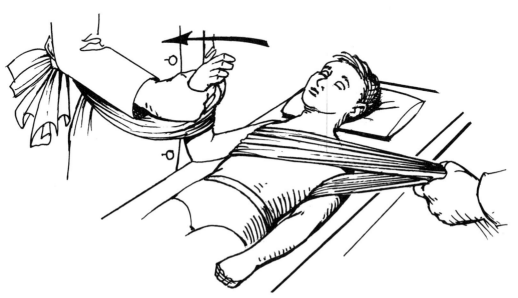

Figure 55–4. Traction–countertraction method for reduction of anterior shoulder dislocation. This technique may require sedation and analgesia.

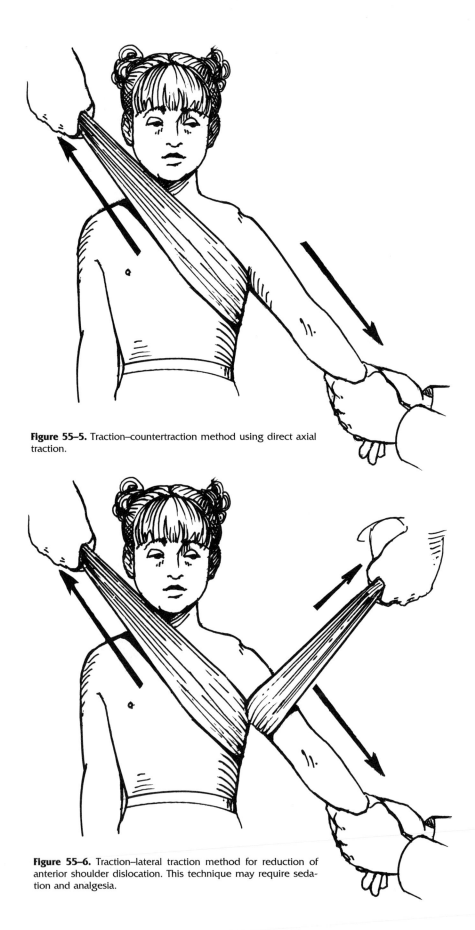

Figure 55–5. Traction–countertraction method using direct axial traction.

Figure 55–6. Traction–lateral traction method for reduction of anterior shoulder dislocation. This technique may require sedation and analgesia.

7. Post reduction care should include radiographs, reassessment of neurovascular function, and the application of a sling and swath.

NOTE: The traction-countertraction and traction-lateral traction methods are usually reserved for dislocations that fail to reduce with either Hennepin's or Stimson's techniques. Both are likely to require systemic analgesia and/or sedation.

Traction–Lateral Traction

1. Confirm the diagnosis of anterior shoulder dislocation, and the absence of an associated fracture with radiographs. Consider sedation and analgesia.
2. This method is similar to the traction-countertraction technique described earlier. The patient is placed in a supine position on a gurney, with countertraction applied via a sheet tied around the upper chest and under the axilla of the affected shoulder.
3. A second sheet is wrapped around the upper arm of the affected extremity and gentle lateral traction is applied (Fig. 55-6).
4. Axial traction is then applied to the extended extremity. If this fails to reduce the dislocation, the extended arm should be slowly adducted across the abdomen, maintaining the axial traction.
5. Post reduction care should include radiographs, reassessment of neurovascular function, and the application of a sling and swath.

COMPLICATIONS

1. Fracture
2. Neurovascular injury (axillary nerve is the most commonly injured)
3. Soft tissue injury (from sheets or straps)

References

Lyman JL, Ervin ME. Management of common dislocations. In Roberts JR, Hedges JR (eds). *Clinical Procedures in Emergency Medicine* (2nd ed). Philadelphia, WB Saunders, 1991.
Ruddy RM (ed). Illustrated techniques of pediatric emergency procedures. In Fleisher GR, Ludwig S (eds). *Textbook of Pediatric Emergency Medicine* (3rd ed). Baltimore, Williams & Wilkins, 1993.
Simon RR, Koenigsknecht SJ. *Emergency Orthopedics—The Extremities* (3rd ed). Norwalk, CT, Appleton and Lange, 1995.

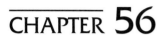

CHAPTER 56

Steven Krug

DISLOCATION REDUCTION—POSTERIOR SHOULDER

INDICATIONS

1. Posterior dislocation of the humeral head
   a. Subacromial: most common type (Fig. 56-1)
   b. Subglenoid
   c. Subspinous
2. The typical findings in patients with a posterior dislocation include blocking of external rotation and limitation of abduction. Patients tend to hold their affected arm in adduction and internal rotation.

CONTRAINDICATIONS

1. Presence of associated fracture to the humeral head or glenoid fossa (these warrant urgent orthopedic consultation)
2. Patients with significant neurovascular compromise of the affected extremity (these too warrant orthopedic consultation)

EQUIPMENT

1. Bedsheets
2. Counterweight
3. Sling and swath

PROCEDURE

NOTE: Posterior dislocations of the shoulder are quite uncommon and generally warrant consultation or specialty referral.

1. Confirm the diagnosis of posterior shoulder dislocation, and the absence of an associated fracture with radiographs. Consider sedation and/or anesthesia.
2. Reduction may be attempted using any of the longitudinal traction techniques

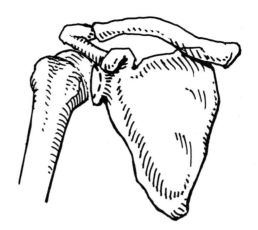

Figure 56–1. Posterior shoulder dislocation.

described for anterior shoulder dislocation (see Figs. 55-2 to 55-6) (see Chapter 55).

3. Post reduction care should include radiographs, reassessment of neurovascular function, and the application of a sling and swath. As posterior dislocations are somewhat uncommon, they all should receive orthopedic referral.

COMPLICATIONS

1. Fracture
2. Neurovascular injury (axillary nerve is most commonly injured)
3. Soft tissue injury (from sheets or straps)

References

Lyman JL, Ervin ME. Management of common dislocations. In Roberts JR, Hedges JR (eds). *Clinical Procedures in Emergency Medicine* (2nd ed). Philadelphia, WB Saunders, 1991.

Ruddy RM (ed). Illustrated techniques of pediatric emergency procedures. In Fleisher GR, Ludwig S (eds). *Textbook of Pediatric Emergency Medicine* (3rd ed). Baltimore, Williams & Wilkins, 1993.

Simon RR, Koenigsknecht SJ. *Emergency Orthopedics—The Extremities* (3rd ed). Norwalk, CT, Appleton and Lange, 1995.

CHAPTER 57

Steven Krug

DISLOCATION REDUCTION—THE ELBOW

INDICATIONS

1. Dislocation (anterior or posterior) of the elbow

NOTE: These injuries are caused by great force and are generally accompanied by associated fractures and significant neurovascular compromise. They warrant urgent orthopedic consultation. The procedures listed here are intended to serve as emergency intervention for patients with a simple dislocation (e.g., no fracture) who have critical neurovascular compromise warranting immediate reduction.

CONTRAINDICATIONS

1. Patients with an associated fracture

EQUIPMENT

1. Equipment and medications necessary for sedation and analgesia. (See Chapter 3.)

PROCEDURES

Posterior Dislocation

1. Confirm the diagnosis of a posterior dislocation and the absence of an associated fracture with radiographs (Fig. 57-1). Conduct a thorough neurovascular examination of the affected extremity.
2. As these injuries are quite painful and are associated with significant muscle spasm, consider the administration of sedation and analgesia.
3. With countertraction applied to the upper arm (typically by an assistant), the physician grasps the wrist and applies steady axial traction with the forearm in a position of supination and slight flexion (Fig. 57-2).
4. If traction alone fails to reduce the joint, continued flexion of the forearm while maintaining traction should serve to cause reduction (Fig. 57-3).
5. Post reduction care includes elevation and a posterior splint (with the elbow at a 90 degree angle) and hospitalization for frequent neurovascular checks.

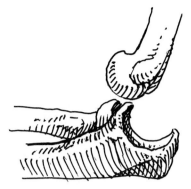

Figure 57–1. Posterior elbow dislocation.

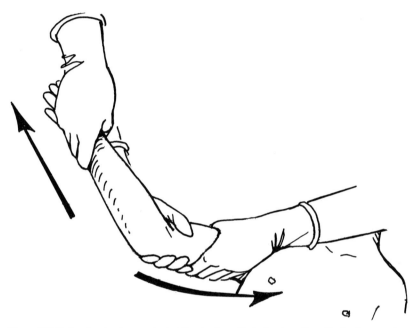

Figure 57–2. Apply steady countertraction to the affected extremity with the forearm in a position of supination and slight flexion. Usually this requires sedation and analgesia.

Figure 57–3. Continued flexion of the forearm while maintaining traction may be necessary to cause reduction.

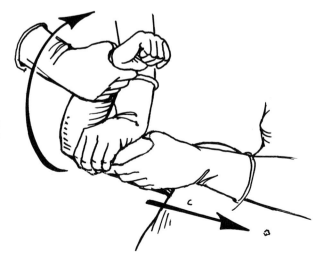

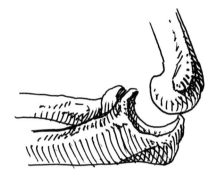

Figure 57–4. Anterior dislocation of the elbow.

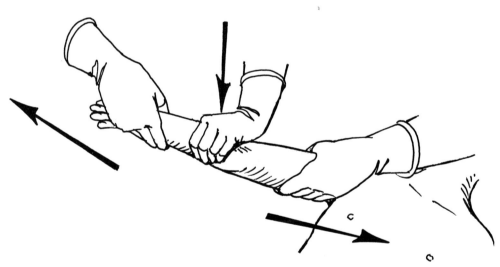

Figure 57–5. With steady countertraction applied to the affected extremity, a downward force is applied to the proximal radius and ulna. This procedure will probably require sedation and analgesia.

Anterior Dislocation

1. Confirm the diagnosis of a posterior dislocation and the absence of an associated fracture with radiographs (Fig. 57-4). Conduct a thorough neurovascular examination of the affected extremity.
2. As these injuries are quite painful and are associated with significant muscle spasm, consider the administration of sedation and analgesia.
3. With countertraction applied to the upper arm by an assistant, the physician grasps the wrist and applies steady axial traction with one hand while the other is used to apply a steady downward force on the proximal radius and ulna (Fig. 57-5).
4. Post reduction care includes elevation and a posterior splint (with the elbow at a 45-degree angle) and hospitalization for frequent neurovascular checks.

COMPLICATIONS

1. Fracture
2. Neurovascular injury
3. Soft tissue injury
4. Compartment syndrome
5. Traumatic myositis ossificans

References

Lyman JL, Ervin ME. Management of common dislocations. In Roberts JR, Hedges JR (eds). *Clinical Procedures in Emergency Medicine* (2nd ed). Philadelphia, WB Saunders, 1991.

Ruddy RM (ed). Illustrated techniques of pediatric emergency procedures. In Fleisher GR, Ludwig S (eds). *Textbook of Pediatric Emergency Medicine* (3rd ed). Baltimore, Williams & Wilkins, 1993.

Simon RR, Koenigsknecht SJ. *Emergency Orthopedics—The Extremities,* (3rd ed). Norwalk, CT, Appleton & Lange, 1995.

CHAPTER 58

Steven Krug

DISLOCATION REDUCTION—THE FINGER

INDICATIONS

1. Simple dorsal dislocation of the thumb or fingers, typically the proximal interphalangeal joint

CONTRAINDICATIONS

1. Presence of an associated fracture in or adjacent to the articular surfaces
2. Complex dislocation: In this type of dislocation, the volar plate has been avulsed and is interposed between the joint surfaces. This type of dislocation can be reduced only with an operative technique.
3. Metacarpophalangeal dislocations: These are typically complex dislocations or are associated with fractures.

EQUIPMENT

1. Equipment and medications necessary for a digital block. (See Chapter 40.)

PROCEDURES

Proximal Interphalangeal Joint

1. Confirm the diagnosis of a dislocation (Fig. 58–1) and the absence of an associated fracture with radiographs. Conduct a thorough neurovascular examination of the affected extremity.
2. Provide a digital block for the affected finger.
3. Grasping the injured digit with one hand, apply gentle axial traction while providing countertraction with the other hand. The key is to provide as little traction as is necessary to reduce the dislocation. Simple traction alone may cause relocation.
4. While applying in-line traction, the digit is slightly hyperextended distal to the dislocation while the base of the dislocated phalanx is pushed downward (Fig. 58–2).

Figure 58–1. Dislocation of proximal interphalangeal joint.

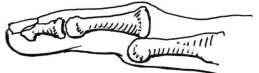

5. If the digit fails to reduce, one must assume that it is a complex dislocation and obtain orthopedic consultation.
6. Post reduction care should include a thorough evaluation for joint instability and splinting of the joint in a position of flexion (15 to 20 degrees). Orthopedic referral is highly recommended for all finger dislocations.

Distal Interphalangeal Joint

1. Confirm the diagnosis of a dislocation and the absence of an associated fracture with radiographs. Conduct a painstaking neurovascular examination of the affected extremity.
2. Provide a digital block for the affected finger.
3. Grasping the injured digit with one hand, apply gentle axial traction while providing countertraction with the other hand (Fig. 58-3). The key is to provide as little traction as necessary to reduce the dislocation. Simple dislocations of this joint usually reduce easily.
4. If the digit fails to reduce, assume it is a complex dislocation and obtain orthopedic consultation.
5. Post reduction care should include a thorough evaluation for joint instability and splinting of the joint in a position of full extension. Orthopedic referral is highly recommended for all finger dislocations.

Figure 58–2. Slight hyperextension of the digit while applying in-line traction usually reduces proximal interphalangeal or metacarpophalangeal dislocations.

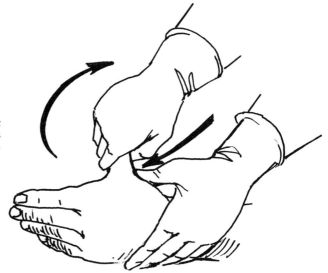

Figure 58–3. Reduction of distal interphalangeal joint dislocation.

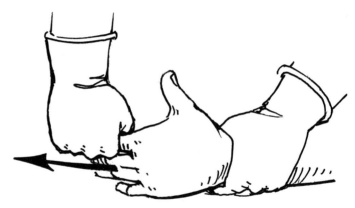
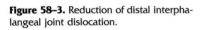

COMPLICATIONS

1. Fracture
2. Neurovascular injury
3. Soft tissue injury

References

Lyman JL, Ervin ME. Management of common dislocations. In Roberts JR, Hedges JR (eds). *Clinical Procedures in Emergency Medicine* (2nd ed). Philadelphia, WB Saunders, 1991.

Ruddy RM (ed). Illustrated techniques of pediatric emergency procedures. In Fleisher GR, Ludwig S (eds). *Textbook of Pediatric Emergency Medicine* (3rd ed). Baltimore, Williams & Wilkins, 1993.

Simon RR, Koenigsknecht SJ. *Emergency Orthopedics—The Extremities* (3rd ed). Norwalk, CT, Appleton & Lange, 1995.

CHAPTER 59

Steven Krug

DISLOCATION REDUCTION—THE HIP

INDICATIONS

1. Dislocation of the femoral head

NOTE: Acute hip dislocation is a very unusual injury in children. Typically, a great amount of force is necessary to dislocate this very stable joint. While preferably treated by an orthopedic surgeon and in an operating room setting with deep or general anesthesia, these injuries must be treated rather quickly to prevent serious complications such as avascular femoral necrosis. In caring for these patients, consideration should be given to the potential for other injuries.

CONTRAINDICATIONS

1. Presence of an associated fracture of the joint surface

EQUIPMENT

1. Equipment and medications necessary for sedation and analgesia. (See Chapter 3.)

PROCEDURE

Posterior Dislocation—Stimson's Technique

1. Confirm the diagnosis of a dislocation (Fig. 59-1) and the absence of an associated fracture with radiographs. Conduct a thorough neurovascular examination of the affected extremity.
2. As these injuries are quite painful and are associated with significant muscle spasm, consider the administration of sedation and analgesia.
3. The patient is placed in a prone position on an examining table or gurney with the hips positioned at the edge of the surface and the affected leg hanging off the bed. An assistant should stabilize the hips.
4. The knee of the injured extremity is flexed to 90 degrees and steady downward traction applied by the physician to the calf just distal to the knee. This may be continued for 10 to 20 min (Fig. 59-2).

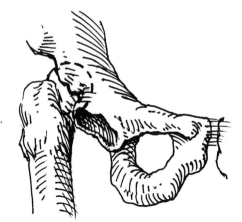

Figure 59–1. Posterior dislocation of the hip.

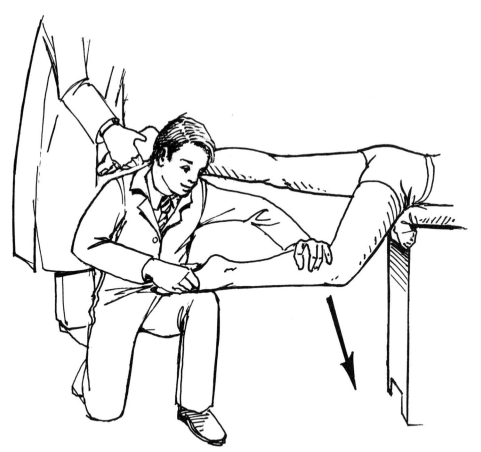

Figure 59–2. Stimson technique for reduction of posterior hip dislocation. This procedure will require sedation and anesthesia.

NOTE: Much like Stimson's technique for shoulder reduction, a hanging weight may be used. (See Chapter 55.)

5. While downward traction is applied, gentle pressure is applied over the greater trocanter, easing it into the acetabulum.
6. Post reduction care includes radiographs to confirm joint relocation (and the absence of fractures) and hospitalization for inline skin traction.

Anterior Dislocation

1. Confirm the diagnosis of a dislocation (Fig. 59-3) and the absence of an associated fracture with radiographs. Conduct a thorough neurovascular examination of the affected extremity.
2. As these injuries are quite painful and are associated with significant muscle spasm, consider the administration of sedation and analgesia.
3. The patient should be placed in a supine position. The pelvis should be held steady by an assistant.
4. With the hip and knee joints each flexed at 90 degrees, the femur should be rotated to a neutral or midline position (Fig. 59-4).
5. One should then apply steady in-line traction to the femur (countertraction is provided by the assistant holding the patient over the iliac crest), with the hands placed on the calf just proximal to the knee (Fig. 59-4). If this fails to reduce the dislocation, the addition of mild internal rotation should help to do so.

NOTE: Adduction of the femur prior to relocation of the femoral head in the acetabulum may result in a fracture of the femoral head or neck.

6. Once the dislocation is reduced, while maintaining traction on the femur, the knee is gradually extended and the leg is lowered to the gurney (Fig. 59-5).
7. Post reduction care includes radiographs to confirm joint relocation (and the absence of fractures) and hospitalization for in-line skin traction.

COMPLICATIONS

1. Fracture—Femoral head or neck
2. Avascular necrosis of the femoral head
3. Neurovascular injury—Sciatic nerve most commonly injured
4. Soft tissue injury

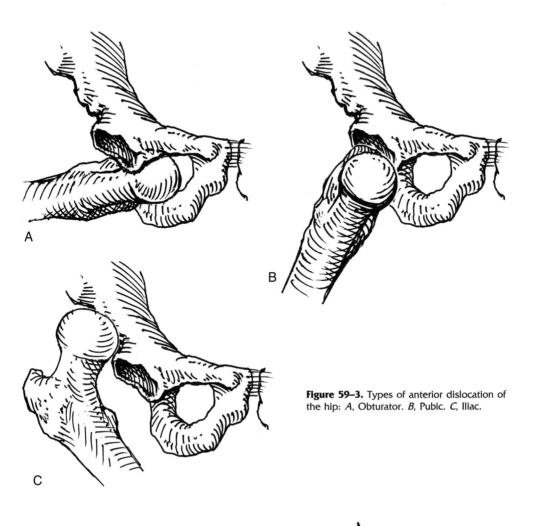

Figure 59–3. Types of anterior dislocation of the hip: *A*, Obturator. *B*, Pubic. *C*, Iliac.

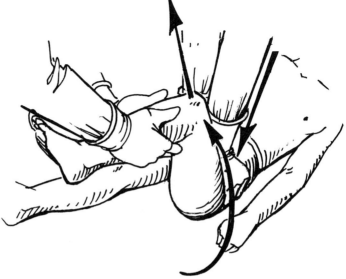

Figure 59–4. Steady in-line traction must be applied to the femur while rotating it into a midline position with the hip and knee flexed at 90 degrees. This procedure requires sedation and analgesia for success.

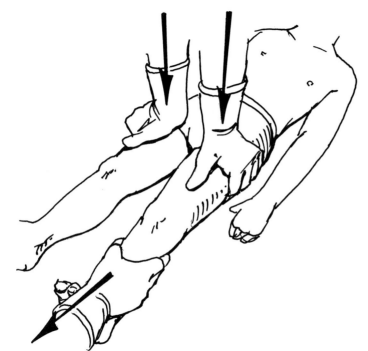

Figure 59–5. Once the hip dislocation is reduced, the knee is gradually extended while maintaining traction on the femur.

References

Lyman JL, Ervin ME. Management of common dislocations. In Roberts JR, Hedges JR (eds). *Clinical Procedures in Emergency Medicine* (2nd ed). Philadelphia, WB Saunders, 1991.

Ruddy RM (ed). Illustrated techniques of pediatric emergency procedures. In Fleisher GR, Ludwig S (eds). *Textbook of Pediatric Emergency Medicine* (3rd ed). Baltimore, Williams & Wilkins, 1993.

Simon RR, Koenigsknecht SJ. *Emergency Orthopedics—The Extremities* (3rd ed). Norwalk, CT, Appleton & Lange, 1995.

CHAPTER 60

Steven Krug

DISLOCATION REDUCTION—THE KNEE

INDICATIONS

1. Dislocation of the knee
   a. Anterior (Fig. 60-1*A*) (most common)
   b. Posterior (Fig. 60-1*B*)
   c. Lateral
   d. Medial

NOTE: Knee dislocations are typically associated with significant ligamentous injury and injury to neurovascular structures. Although they warrant urgent reduction in order to minimize the risk for permanent neurovascular injury, they are best reduced in an operating room setting with deep or general anesthesia. Emergency department reduction should be attempted only in the presence of significant neurovascular compromise that can be reversible with reduction and when specialty consultation is not immediately available.

CONTRAINDICATIONS

1. Presence of an associated fracture of the joint surface

EQUIPMENT

1. Equipment and medications necessary for sedation and analgesia. (See Chapter 3.)

PROCEDURE

1. Confirm the diagnosis of a dislocation and the absence of an associated fracture with radiographs. Conduct a thorough neurovascular examination of the affected extremity.
2. As these injuries are quite painful and are associated with significant muscle spasm, consider the administration of sedation and analgesia.
3. The patient is placed in a supine position. Stabilization of the thigh (and countertraction) are applied by one assistant while another provides steady axial traction on the lower leg (Fig. 60-2).

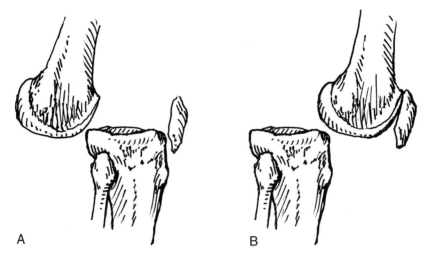

Figure 60–1. Dislocation of the knee. *A,* Anterior. *B,* Posterior.

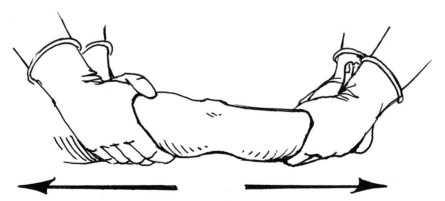

Figure 60–2. Reduction of knee dislocation requires steady traction–countertraction of the affected extremity. This procedure typically requires sedation and analgesia.

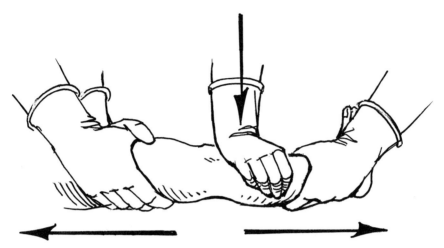

Figure 60–3. With traction–countertraction applied, gentle downward pressure applied to the proximal tibia will relocate an anterior dislocation.

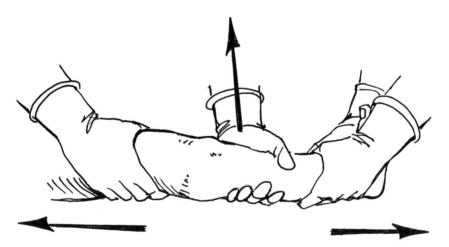

Figure 60–4. With traction–countertraction applied, the posteriorly dislocated tibia should be lifted over the distal femur.

4. With traction-countertraction applied, the physician relocates the joint as follows:
   a. Anterior dislocation: The physician places gentle downward pressure over the proximal tibia, while gently pulling upward on the distal third of the femur (Fig. 60-3).
   b. Posterior dislocation: The posteriorly displaced tibia is gently lifted over the distal femur and into place (Fig. 60-4).
   c. Lateral dislocation: The laterally displaced tibia is gently lifted over the lateral femoral condyle and into the joint space. This may be facilitated by placing the knee in 60 to 90 degrees of flexion.
   d. Medial dislocation: The medially displaced tibia is gently lifted over the medial femoral condyle and into the joint space. This may be facilitated by placing the knee in 60 to 90 degrees of flexion.

COMPLICATIONS

1. Fracture: tibial plateau, femoral condyles, patella
2. Neurovascular injury
3. Soft tissue injury

References

Lyman JL, Ervin ME. Management of common dislocations. In Roberts JR, Hedges JR (eds). *Clinical Procedures in Emergency Medicine* (2nd ed). Philadelphia, WB Saunders, 1991.

Ruddy RM (ed). Illustrated techniques of pediatric emergency procedures. In Fleisher GR, Ludwig S (eds). *Textbook of Pediatric Emergency Medicine* (3rd ed). Baltimore, Williams & Wilkins, 1993.

Simon RR, Koenigsknecht SJ. *Emergency Orthopedics—The Extremities* (3rd ed). Norwalk, CT, Appleton and Lange, 1995.

CHAPTER 61

Steven Krug

DISLOCATION REDUCTION—THE PATELLA

INDICATIONS

1. Dislocation of the patella
   A. Lateral (the most common type), usually amenable to closed reduction
   B. Medial, superior, intra-articular (these are rare), very difficult to reduce and typically require operative intervention

CONTRAINDICATIONS

1. Presence of an associated fracture of the patella or the joint surface

EQUIPMENT

1. Equipment and medications as necessary for sedation and analgesia. (See Chapter 3.)

PROCEDURES

Lateral Dislocation

1. Confirm the diagnosis of a dislocation and the absence of an associated fracture with radiographs. Conduct a thorough neurovascular examination of the affected extremity.
2. While these injuries can be quite painful and are associated with significant muscle spasm, the patella can usually be reduced without parenteral analgesia. Still, one should consider the benefits of the administration of sedation and analgesia.
3. The patient is placed in a supine or sitting position. The knee is slowly extended to 180 degrees. Extension alone is commonly all that is needed to relocate the patella.
4. If extension fails to relocate the patella, the application of a gentle downward and medial force to the lateral aspect of the patella should allow the medial border of the patella to move over the lateral femoral condyle and into position (Fig. 61-1).

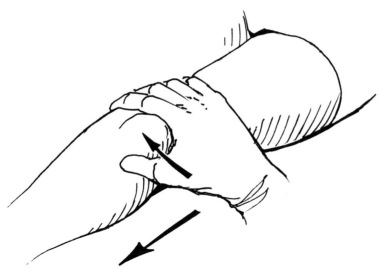

Figure 61–1. If extension of the leg fails to relocate the patella, the application of a downward and medial force should move the patella into position.

5. Post reduction care includes radiographs to confirm patella relocation and the absence of fractures. The patient should be placed in a knee immobilizer.

COMPLICATIONS

1. Fracture
2. Neurovascular injury
3. Soft tissue injury

References

Lyman JL, Ervin ME. Management of common dislocations. In Roberts JR, Hedges JR (eds). *Clinical Procedures in Emergency Medicine* (2nd ed). Philadelphia, WB Saunders, 1991.
Ruddy RM (ed). Illustrated techniques of pediatric emergency procedures. In Fleisher GR, Ludwig S (eds). *Textbook of Pediatric Emergency Medicine* (3rd ed). Baltimore, Williams & Wilkins, 1993.
Simon RR, Koenigsknecht SJ. *Emergency Orthopedics—The Extremities* (3rd ed). Norwalk, CT, Appleton & Lange, 1995.

CHAPTER 62

Steven Krug

DISLOCATION REDUCTION—THE ANKLE

INDICATIONS

1. Dislocation of the distal fibula and tibia
   a. Anterior (Fig. 62-1*A*)
   b. Posterior (Fig. 62-1*B*) (most common)

NOTE: Ankle dislocations are typically associated with significant force and ligamentous injury and fractures.

CONTRAINDICATIONS

1. Presence of an associated fracture of the joint surface

EQUIPMENT

1. Equipment and medications necessary for sedation and analgesia. (See Chapter 3.)

PROCEDURE

Posterior Dislocation

1. Confirm the diagnosis of a dislocation and the absence of an associated fracture with radiographs. Conduct a thorough neurovascular examination of the affected extremity.
2. As these injuries are quite painful and are associated with significant muscle spasm, consider the administration of sedation and analgesia.
3. Place the patient in a supine position, with the knee of the injured leg in a position of flexion.
4. With an assistant providing countertraction on the mid-calf, the examiner should apply axial traction. One hand supports the foot at the heel and the other holds the forefoot in a position of plantar flexion (Fig. 62-2).
5. While maintaining countertraction, a second assistant provides downward counter-pressure on the anterior surface of the lower leg. The examiner should then

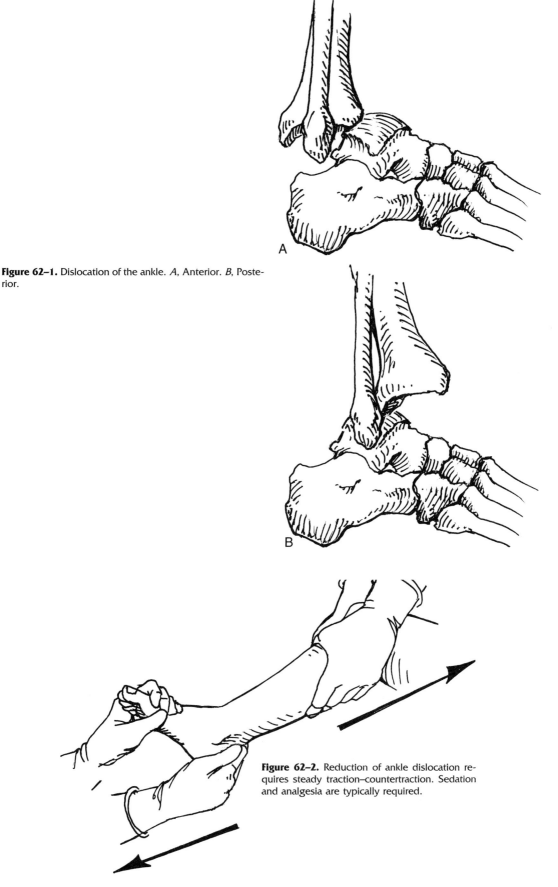

Figure 62–1. Dislocation of the ankle. *A*, Anterior. *B*, Posterior.

Figure 62–2. Reduction of ankle dislocation requires steady traction–countertraction. Sedation and analgesia are typically required.

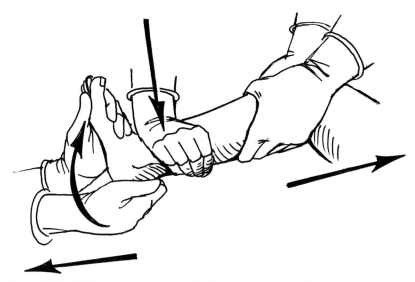

Figure 62–3. With constant traction applied, the posteriorly dislocated foot should be lifted anteriorly in a dorsiflexed position.

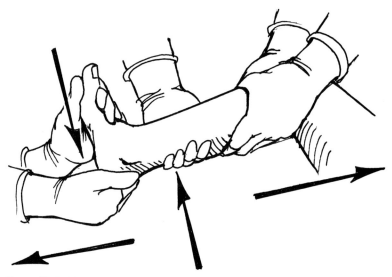

Figure 62–4. With constant traction applied, the anteriorly dislocated foot is pushed downward while the assistant lifts the distal calf.

apply upward traction and gently dorsiflex the foot, pulling the foot forward into a neutral position (Fig. 62–3).
6. Post reduction care includes radiographs to confirm joint relocation (and the absence of fractures), splinting the ankle in a neutral position, and hospitalization with frequent reassessment for neurovascular integrity.

Anterior Dislocation

1. Confirm the diagnosis of a dislocation and the absence of an associated fracture with radiographs. Conduct a thorough neurovascular examination of the affected extremity.
2. As these injuries are quite painful and are associated with significant muscle spasm, consider the administration of sedation and analgesia.
3. The patient is placed in a supine position with the knee slightly flexed. Axial traction should be applied by grasping the foot with both hands while an assistant provides countertraction on the calf (see Fig. 62–2).
4. While traction is maintained, the foot is further dorsiflexed while a second assistant grasps the underside of the distal calf and lifts upward; the physician simultaneously pushes the foot in a posterior direction (Fig. 62–4).
5. Post reduction care includes radiographs to confirm joint relocation (and the absence of fractures), splinting of the ankle in a neutral position, and hospitalization with frequent reassessment for neurovascular integrity.

COMPLICATIONS

1. Fracture
2. Avascular necrosis of the talus
3. Neurovascular injury
4. Soft tissue injury

References

Lyman JL, Ervin ME. Management of common dislocations. In Roberts JR, Hedges JR (eds). *Clinical Procedures in Emergency Medicine* (2nd ed). Philadelphia, WB Saunders, 1991.
Ruddy RM (ed). Illustrated techniques of pediatric emergency procedures. In Fleisher GR, Ludwig S (eds). *Textbook of Pediatric Emergency Medicine* (3rd ed). Baltimore, Williams & Wilkins, 1993.
Simon RR, Koenigsknecht SJ. *Emergency Orthopedics—The Extremities* (3rd ed). Norwalk, CT, Appleton & Lange, 1995.

OPHTHALMOLOGY/ OTOLARYNGOLOGY

CHAPTER 63

Steven Krug

EYE PATCHING

INDICATIONS

1. Corneal injury (blunt trauma, chemical or ultraviolet radiation injury)

CONTRAINDICATIONS

1. Corneal ulcer
2. Penetrating eye trauma

EQUIPMENT

1. Gauze eye patches, two or more
2. Tape
3. Ophthalmologic antibiotic ointment
4. Gloves

PROCEDURE

1. Instill antibiotic ointment in eye to be patched.

NOTE: You may also want to consider instilling a cycloplegic agent, particularly for patients who have suffered blunt trauma to the eye.

2. Have patient close both eyes and keep them so until the completion of the procedure.
3. Fold the first patch in half and place over the closed lids.
4. Place the second patch, unfolded, in a horizontal position over the first (Fig. 63-1). A third patch can be placed over the second patch in a similar manner. The patch must be bulky enough to prevent opening of the eye.
5. Place tape diagonally over the patch running from the mid-forehead to the cheek (Fig. 63-2).

NOTE: The patch should not be left in place for more than 24 hr.

COMPLICATIONS

1. Corneal abrasion
2. Pain and delayed healing (usually caused by a loose patch)
3. Recurrent corneal erosions

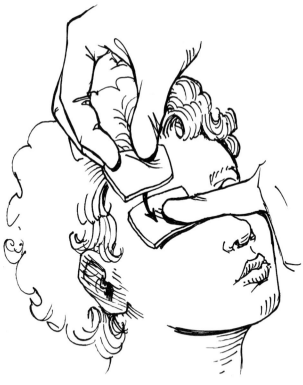

Figure 63–1. Application of eye patch. The patch must be bulky enough to prevent opening of the eye.

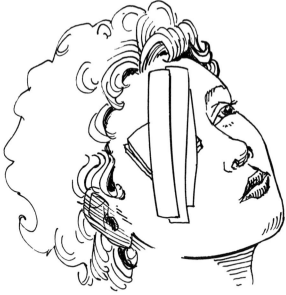

Figure 63–2. Recommended taping of eye patch.

References

Barr DH, Samples JR, Hedges JR. Ophthalmologic procedures. In Roberts JR, Hedges JR (eds). *Clinical Procedures in Emergency Medicine* (2nd ed). Philadelphia, WB Saunders, 1991.

Ruddy RM (ed). Illustrated techniques of pediatric emergency procedures. In Fleisher GR, Ludwig S (eds). *Textbook of Pediatric Emergency Medicine* (3rd ed). Baltimore, Williams & Wilkins, 1993.

CHAPTER 64

Steven Krug

EYELID EVERSION AND RETRACTION

INDICATIONS

1. Examination of the anterior surface of the eye
2. Location and removal of a foreign body

CONTRAINDICATIONS

1. Suspected rupture or laceration of the globe

EQUIPMENT

1. Cotton swab
2. Desmarres lid retractor(s)
3. Gloves
4. Topical ophthalmologic anesthetic—0.5 to 1.0% tetracaine or 0.5% proparacaine

PROCEDURES

Lid Eversion

1. With the child well restrained, grasp the lashes of the upper lid between the thumb and index finger of the dominant hand. Pull the eyelid downward.
2. Place a cotton swap on the upper lid at the superior tarsal margin (Fig. 64-1*A*).
3. Move the swab downward as the eyelid is then pulled slowly upward. This should cause bending or rolling back of the eyelid onto the swab, exposing the palpebral surface (Fig. 64-1*B*).
4. Lifting the swab away from the surface of the lid while maintaining slight pressure along the lid margin should reverse the procedure.
5. The same procedure can be used for the lower lid, although the lower lid can usually be easily everted using the fingers alone by placing the thumb and index finger at the base of the lid and retracting in a caudal direction (Fig. 64-2).

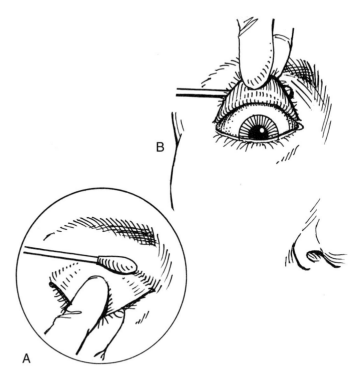

Figure 64–1. Eyelid eversion. *A,* Cotton swab placed on the upper lid at the tarsal margin. *B,* Pulling swab downward as eyelid is pulled upward should evert the lid.

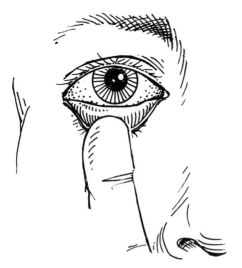

Figure 64–2. Eversion of lower eyelid.

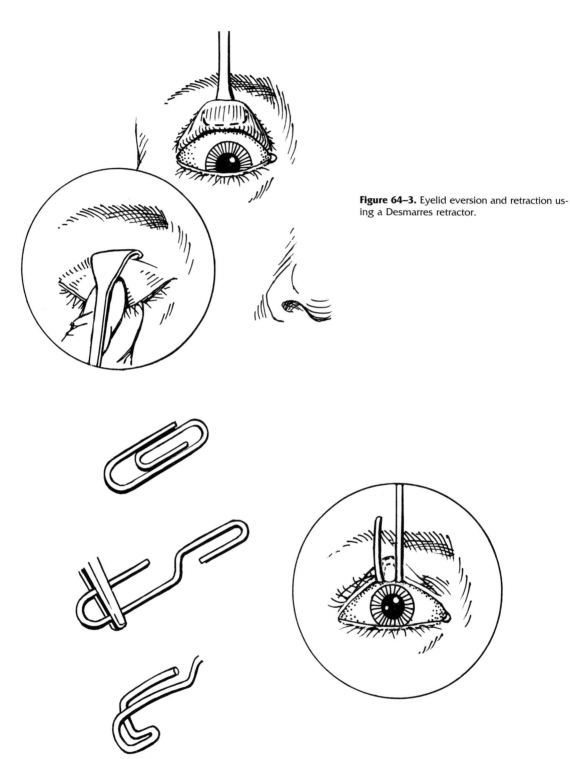

Figure 64–3. Eyelid eversion and retraction using a Desmarres retractor.

Figure 64–4. Standard paper clip fashioned into a lid retractor.

Lid Retraction

1. This is the preferred technique for exposing the eye when there is concern for the presence of penetrating injury or a traumatic rupture.
2. Instill 1 drop of topical anesthetic into the eye.
3. Using the same technique described for eyelid eversion, and a Desmarres retractor, one can both evert and retract the upper lid (Fig. 64-3). This technique provides for a great deal of exposure of the globe. The Desmarres retractor can also be used by simply slipping it between the lid and the globe and manually retracting the lid.
4. If a commercial retractor is not available, a paper clip can be fashioned into a retractor by using a hemostat (Fig. 64-4).
5. If prolonged retraction of the lids is anticipated, one may wish to use a lid speculum.

COMPLICATIONS

1. Trauma to the lid
2. Infection (conjunctivitis)
3. Corneal abrasion

References

Barr DH, Samples JR, Hedges JR. Ophthalmologic procedures. In Roberts JR, Hedges JR (eds). *Clinical Procedures in Emergency Medicine* (2nd ed). Philadelphia, WB Saunders, 1991.
Ruddy RM (ed). Illustrated techniques of pediatric emergency procedures. In Fleisher GR, Ludwig S (eds). *Textbook of Pediatric Emergency Medicine* (3rd ed). Baltimore, Williams & Wilkins, 1993.

CHAPTER 65

Steven Krug

FOREIGN BODY REMOVAL—EYE

INDICATIONS

1. Presence of external or extraocular foreign body
2. Clinical suspicion of ocular foreign body

CONTRAINDICATIONS

1. Suspected penetrating eye injury or ruptured globe
2. Embedded foreign body—whereas the removal of an embedded corneal or conjunctival foreign body may be attempted in adult patients, it is recommended that children with such injuries receive ophthalmologic consultation.

EQUIPMENT

1. Ophthalmoscope or slit lamp
2. Topical anesthetic (0.5 to 1.0% tetracaine, 0.5% proparacaine)
3. Eyelid retractors
4. Sterile cotton-tipped applicators
5. Wood's lamp
6. Fluorescein strips or drops
7. Ophthalmologic antibiotic ointment
8. Eye patches and tape
9. Gloves

PROCEDURE

1. Perform a careful screening eye examination to rule out an intraocular foreign body (e.g., a penetrating injury). If this is suspected, apply an eye shield and obtain urgent consultation with an ophthalmologist.
2. Apply a drop of topical anesthetic; this will assist the examination.
3. Attempt to locate the foreign body by examining the surface of the globe and the undersides of each lid (see Chapter 64). As plain vision will not uncover small foreign objects, this examination should be assisted by a slit lamp or ophthalmoscope.

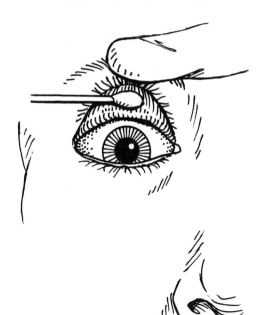

Figure 65–1. Removal of a conjunctival foreign body. This can be done using a cotton-tipped applicator.

4. If a foreign body is located, attempt removal with a cotton-tipped applicator (Fig. 65-1). Very tiny objects may be best removed with a nasopharyngeal swab or Calgiswab. If the foreign body fails to move, it is likely embedded.

NOTE: A very superficial embedded foreign body may be removed with the assistance of an "eye spud" or a 25- or 27-gauge needle. This procedure risks penetrating injury to the eye and should be attempted only in the cooperative patient by an experienced practitioner.

5. If the foreign body is not located, apply fluorescein to the eye and reexamine for the presence of abrasions. Certain small foreign bodies may have an area of intense staining around them. Others may be located by following the track of a linear abrasion, especially so under the eyelid.
6. Upon completion of the examination (and removal of the foreign body if present), antibiotic ointment should be instilled and the eye patched (see Chapter 63).

COMPLICATIONS

1. Missed foreign body or incomplete removal
2. Corneal or conjunctival abrasion
3. Conjunctivitis
4. Globe penetration

References

Barr DH, Samples JR, Hedges JR. Ophthalmologic procedures. In Roberts JR, Hedges JR (eds). *Clinical Procedures in Emergency Medicine* (2nd ed). Philadelphia, WB Saunders, 1991.
Ruddy RM (ed). Illustrated techniques of pediatric emergency procedures. In Fleisher GR, Ludwig S (eds). *Textbook of Pediatric Emergency Medicine* (3rd ed). Baltimore, Williams & Wilkins, 1993.

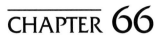

Steven Krug

CONTACT LENS REMOVAL

INDICATIONS

1. Presence of contact lens in patient with altered mental status
2. Presence of contact lens in patient with eye trauma

CONTRAINDICATION

1. Suspected penetrating injury or ruptured globe

EQUIPMENT

1. Suction-tipped contact lens removal device
2. Gloves

PROCEDURES

Hard Lens

1. In the cooperative patient who can sit upright, manually retract the eyelids on the lateral aspect of the palpebral margin. Instruct the patient to look toward his or her nose and then downward toward the chin. This will serve to move the lower lid margin under the lens and cause it to be flipped off the eye.
2. In the uncooperative or supine patient, the simplest technique for lens removal is to use a moistened suction-tipped device to remove the lens from the eye surface (Fig. 66–1).
3. If a suction device is not available, the lens may be removed as follows:
   a. One thumb is placed on each lid near the lid margin and the lids are retracted well beyond the margins of the lens (Fig. 66–2A).
   b. The lids are then pressed firmly against the globe and the lid margins are gently advanced to the borders of the lens (Fig. 66–2B).
   c. The lower lid is pressed so that it moves under the lower edge of the lens.
   d. The lids are slowly closed, allowing the lens to flip off the eye (Fig. 66–2C).

NOTE: This technique should not be used in patients with a suspected penetrating eye injury.

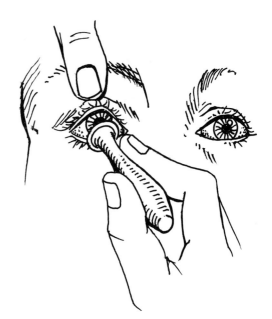

Figure 66–1. Removal of hard contact lens using suction-tipped device.

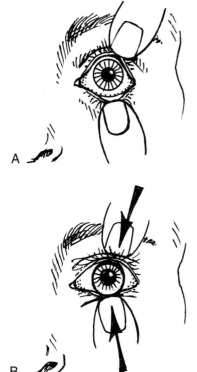

A

B

Figure 66–2. Removal of hard contact lens. *A*, Retraction of eyelids. *B*, Lids are pressed firmly against the globe with lid margins advanced to borders of lens. *C*, Lids are closed, allowing the lens to flip off the eye.

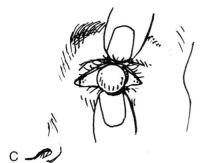

C

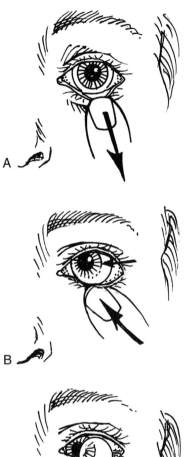

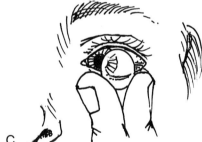

Figure 66–3. Removal of soft contact lens. *A*, Retract lower eyelid. *B*, Slide lens off cornea onto conjunctiva. *C*, Grasp lens by pinching between thumb and forefinger.

Soft Lens

1. Retract the lower eyelid using the middle finger (Fig. 66-3*A*).
2. Slide the lens off the cornea onto the sclera using the index finger (Fig. 66-3*B*).
3. Pinch the lens between the index finger and the thumb. This should allow for removal of the lens from the eye (Fig. 66-3*C*).
4. If the previous steps fail or are poorly tolerated by the patient, a soft lens suction-tipped removal device should be considered.

COMPLICATIONS

1. Corneal abrasion
2. Conjunctivitis
3. Further injury to a ruptured globe

References

Barr DH, Samples JR, Hedges JR. Ophthalmologic procedures. In Roberts JR, Hedges JR (eds). *Clinical Procedures in Emergency Medicine* (2nd ed). Philadelphia, WB Saunders, 1991.
Ruddy RM (ed). Illustrated techniques of pediatric emergency procedures. In Fleisher GR, Ludwig S (eds). *Textbook of Pediatric Emergency Medicine* (3rd ed). Baltimore, Williams & Wilkins, 1993.

CHAPTER 67

Steven Krug

EYE IRRIGATION

INDICATIONS

1. Chemical injury to the eye
2. Multiple small extraocular foreign bodies

CONTRAINDICATIONS

1. Suspected penetrating eye injury or globe rupture

EQUIPMENT

1. Topical anesthetic (0.5 to 1.0% tetracaine, 0.5% proparacaine)
2. Lid retractors
3. Irrigating device (e.g., Morgan lens)
4. Irrigation solution (e.g., normal saline)
5. Intravenous (IV) tubing
6. Cotton-tipped applicators
7. Gauze pads
8. pH indicator paper
9. Gloves

PROCEDURE

1. Instill topical analgesic. Consider the use of sedation (see Chapter 3).
2. Retract upper and lower lids and evert upper lid (see Chapter 64). It is recommended that a self-retracting device, such as a Desmarres retractor, be used.
3. Remove any foreign bodies or particulate matter from the surface of the eye and the underside of the lids with a cotton-tipped applicator.
4. Direct a stream of normal saline from the IV tubing into the eye, taking care to avoid direct irrigation onto cornea (this can cause mechanical injury). The fluid should be directed into both the upper and lower fornices (Fig. 67-1*A*, *B*).
5. The duration or amount of irrigation required depends on the cause of the injury:
    a. Acids (with the exception of hydrofluoric and heavy metal acids) are quickly neutralized by eye surface proteins. These generally require only 10 to 20 min of irrigation.
    b. Alkalis (as well as hydrofluoric and heavy metal acids) can penetrate the cornea fairly rapidly and may continue to cause injury for up to 48 hr. These

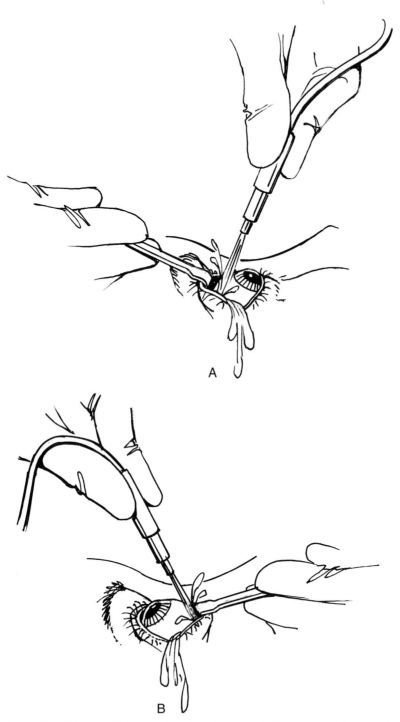

Figure 67–1. Irrigation of the eye. Direction of stream of saline into the following: *A*, Upper fornix. *B*, Lower fornix.

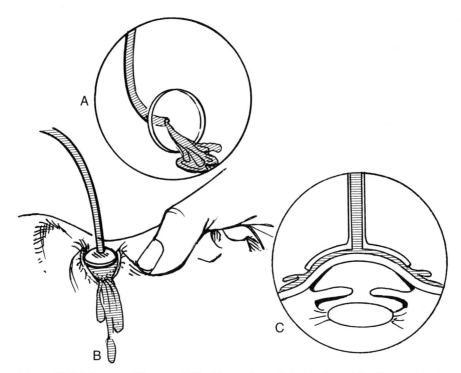

Figure 67–2. Irrigation of the eye. *A*, The Morgan lens. *B*, Application of the Morgan lens to the eye surface. *C*, Cross-sectional view.

injuries require prolonged irrigation. Acutely, these injuries should receive 2 to 4 liters of irrigation over the first hour.

NOTE: All alkali injuries should receive urgent ophthalmologic consultation.

6. As a general guideline, acute irrigation should continue until the pH in the conjunctival fornices has returned to normal (pH = 7.4). This should be re-checked in 15 to 20 min to ensure that it remains normal.
7. As mentioned, alkalis can cause progressive damage to the eye over a period of 48 hr, in spite of aggressive acute irrigation. Patients with alkali injuries are candidates for chronic eye irrigation. This may be accomplished with a Morgan lens or other device (Fig. 67–2).

COMPLICATIONS

1. Abrasion of cornea or conjunctiva

References

Barr DH, Samples JR, Hedges JR. Ophthalmologic procedures. In Roberts JR, Hedges JR (eds). *Clinical Procedures in Emergency Medicine* (2nd ed). Philadelphia, WB Saunders, 1991.
Ruddy RM (ed). Illustrated techniques of pediatric emergency procedures. In Fleisher GR, Ludwig S (eds). *Textbook of Pediatric Emergency Medicine* (3rd ed). Baltimore, Williams & Wilkins, 1993.

CHAPTER 68

Jim R. Harley

OTIC FOREIGN BODY AND CERUMEN REMOVAL

INDICATIONS

1. Presence of a foreign body in the auditory canal
2. Visualization of the tympanic membrane (e.g., cerumen removal)

CONTRAINDICATIONS

1. Perforation of tympanic membrane (irrigation method is contraindicated).

EQUIPMENT

1. Good light source: fiberoptic otoscope, operating otoscope, head lamp, operating microscope with the largest ear speculum that fits.
2. Foreign body removal device: bayonet forceps, alligator forceps, suction-tipped catheter, cerumen ear loop, ear curette, right-angle pick, 20- to 60-ml syringe for irrigation
3. Gloves

PROCEDURES

Mechanical Removal

1. As patient cooperation is important to ensure successful and atraumatic removal, consideration should be given to using sedation and anesthesia.
2. If use of sedation is not an option, one may consider providing a four-quadrant field block for the external canal. This may be accomplished by the subcutaneous injection of 0.3 to 0.5 ml of lidocaine in each of four quadrants encircling the auditory canal (Fig. 68-1*A*).
3. Using a good light source, identify the size, shape, type, and location of the foreign body (Fig. 68-1*B*). These features will help to determine which removal device and technique is best suited.
4. The bayonet forceps or alligator forceps are best used for narrow foreign bodies or those with a small leading edge (Fig. 68-2).

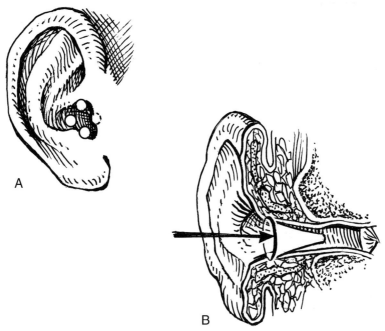

Figure 68–1. Examination of the auditory canal for a foreign body may require sedation, or one of the following: *A*, Local block with subcutaneous lidocaine. *B*, Examination and removal of the foreign body, facilitated by using the largest speculum that will fit.

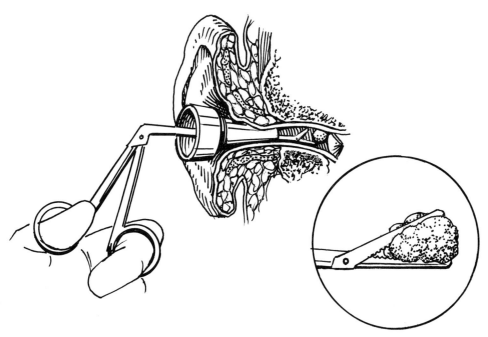

Figure 68–2. Foreign body removal using alligator forceps. Small and narrow objects are best removed by this method.

5. A suction-tipped instrument may be best suited for round, smooth-surfaced objects (Fig. 68–3).

6. An angled wire loop or ear curette can sometimes be placed behind the foreign body, scooping it out of the canal (Fig. 68–4).

7. Certain organic materials, such as beans, may be best removed with a blunt right-angled pick or hook (Fig. 70–2). The object is "punctured" by the tip of the pick and is pulled out of the canal.

Irrigation

1. This technique is especially useful for the removal of small hard objects in the canal. It should be avoided when removing organic material, which may swell when immersed in fluid.

2. Irrigation is best accomplished using a 20- to 60-ml syringe filled with room temperature saline. Either a Silastic vascular catheter (minus the needle) or butterfly needle tubing (with the butterfly needle cut off) will serve well to direct the flow of irrigant into the canal.

3. The patient's head must be positioned to permit the outflow of the irrigant (and the foreign body). Whether the patient is sitting or lying down, the head and the ear canal should be in a neutral position (Fig. 68–5).

Insect Removal

1. The removal of a living insect is a very difficult task. Attempting to remove a live insect will likely result in significant irritation for the patient and the retention and difficult removal of portions of the struggling insect.

2. The first step in the procedure involves suffocation of the insect. This can be accomplished via the instillation of mineral oil or alcohol into the canal.

NOTE: An alternative method is to instill lidocaine in the canal. Lidocaine is very noxious to many insects, and they will find their way out of the canal.

3. Once the insect has been suffocated, it may be removed by either mechanical extraction (alligator forceps, ear loop) or irrigation.

Cerumen Removal

1. Cerumen may be removed using a number of methods, including:
   A. Irrigation (accomplished using a small catheter attached to a syringe, or with a Water Pik).
   B. Suction.
   C. Curettage (using a variety of devices).

2. As irrigation is perhaps the simplest (and potentially the least traumatic), its use is usually the first approach (Fig. 68–5).

NOTE: Irrigation should not be used in children with known or suspected perforation of the tympanic membrane.

3. If irrigation fails, mechanical methods may be required to remove the cerumen.

NOTE: If the cerumen is rather hard and immediate removal is not necessary, it

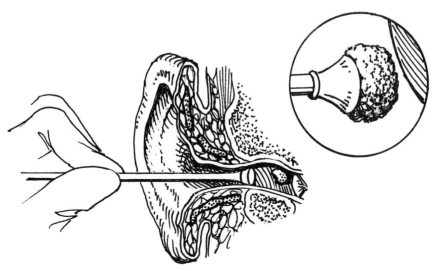

Figure 68–3. Suction-tipped device used to remove round or smooth-surfaced foreign bodies.

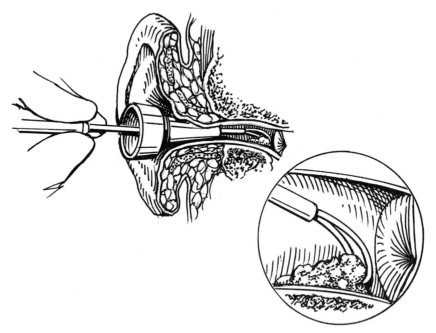

Figure 68–4. Removal of foreign body or cerumen using a wire loop.

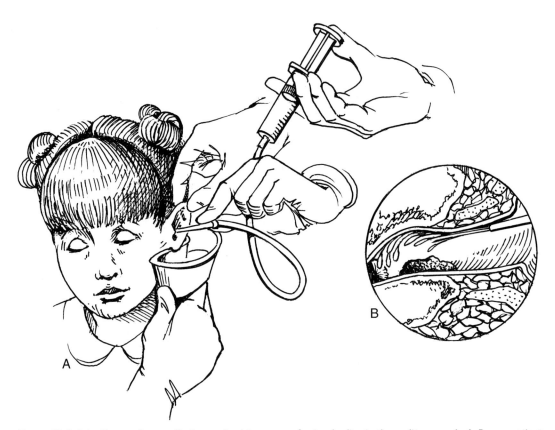

Figure 68–5. Irrigation can be an effective method to remove foreign bodies in the auditory canal. *A*, Proper patient positioning. *B*, Cross-sectional view of the canal.

may be best to recommend that commercial cerumen-softening drops be instilled. The patient can then return for elective removal in 1 to 2 weeks' time.

4. If the cerumen is soft, the best mechanical removal device may be a small Calgiswab. The small size of this swab makes it ideal for especially young infants with narrow canals.
5. For harder cerumen, and in children with larger canals, an ear loop will be required for effective removal (see Fig. 68-4).

COMPLICATIONS

1. Trauma or injury to ear canal
2. Injury to the eardrum or middle ear

References

Abelson TI, Witt WJ. Otolaryngologic procedures. In Roberts JR, Hedges JR (eds). *Clinical Procedures in Emergency Medicine* (2nd ed). Philadelphia, WB Saunders, 1991.
Ruddy RM (ed). Illustrated techniques of pediatric emergency procedures. In Fleisher GR, Ludwig S (eds). *Textbook of Pediatric Emergency Medicine* (3rd ed). Baltimore, Williams & Wilkins, 1993.

CHAPTER 69

Jim R. Harley

NASAL CAUTERY

INDICATIONS

1. Recurrent anterior epistaxis, or anterior epistaxis that fails to remit with 20 to 30 min of direct pressure

CONTRAINDICATIONS

1. Children with clotting disorders: The use of cautery in these patients may simply make the problem worse, because the child may bleed from the lesion created by cautery.

EQUIPMENT

1. Topical anesthetic/vasoconstrictor (2 to 4% lidocaine mixed 50:50 with 0.5% oxymetazoline)

NOTE: Placing a tiny drop of peppermint oil into the 5- to 10-ml mix of lidocaine and oxymetazoline will make the somewhat bitter taste and smell of that mixture much more tolerable for children.

2. Hand-held atomizer or medicine dropper
3. Light source, preferably head lamp
4. Nasal speculum (use the largest size that fits)
5. Cautery device: silver nitrate applicators, heat cautery device
6. Cotton-tipped applicators
7. Normal saline
8. Bayonet forceps
9. Cotton pledgets or cotton balls
10. Gloves

PROCEDURE

1. Have the patient sit, placing the head in a "sniffing" position.
2. Visualize the source of bleeding using the nasal speculum and light source (Fig. 69-1). In order to examine the nasal cavity completely, all blood clots will need to be expelled or removed.
3. Ensure that the bleeding source is indeed the anterior septum (i.e., Little's area) (Fig. 69-2).

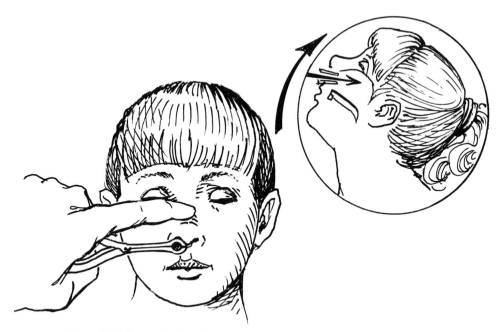

Figure 69–1. Proper hand and patient positioning for nasal speculum examination.

Figure 69–2. Cross-sectional view of the nasal septum. Little's area is the most common source of bleeding in the arterior septum.

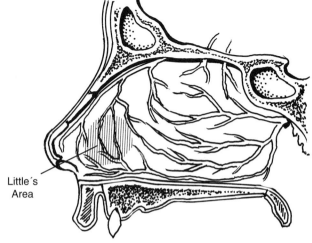

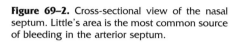

Little´s
Area

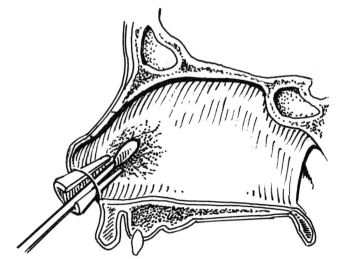

Figure 69–3. Cauterization of anterior nasal septum with silver nitrate.

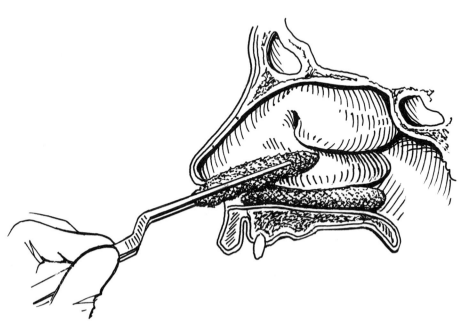

Figure 69–4. Insertion of cotton pledgets with bayonet forceps.

4. Spray or instill topical anesthetic/vasoconstrictor.
5. If bleeding has stopped and the source is identifiable, cautery may be attempted using silver nitrate (Fig. 69-3). Some important tips regarding silver nitrate follow:
   a. Silver nitrate will not work if active bleeding is present.
   b. Use dry cotton-tipped applicators to keep the cautery area as dry as possible.
   c. To be effective, the silver nitrate must be held on the mucosa for 10 to 15 sec.
   d. Do not allow silver nitrate–laden secretions to drip back into the airway, as they will cause caustic injury.
   e. Do not allow silver nitrate–laden secretions to run out of the nose onto the face, as they will cause skin discoloration.
   f. Saline moistened cotton-tipped applicators should be used to neutralize and remove excess silver nitrate.
6. If bleeding has not stopped with spray application of lidocaine/oxymetazoline, one can try direct application of that agent using a cotton pledget. The pledget, which can be made by making an elongated roll of a cotton ball, should be soaked in lidocaine/oxymetazoline.
7. The pledget is inserted using a nasal speculum and a bayonet forceps. It should be applied directly to the bleeding site and held firmly in place for 5 min (Fig. 69-4).
8. If this fails, one may consider using 4% cocaine solution (not the 10% solution) as the topical anesthetic/vasoconstrictor, either sprayed on the mucosa or applied directly with a pledget.

NOTE: Children with bleeding disorders frequently require cocaine (rather than lidocaine/oxymetazoline) for effective vasoconstriction and hemostasis. Cocaine must be used with great caution when applied to mucous membranes.

9. If bleeding is stopped with the pledget, remove the pledget and proceed with silver nitrate cautery.
10. If bleeding cannot be stopped, heat cautery may be attempted. Generally, if chemical cautery fails, proceed with nasal packing and obtain otolaryngology consultation (see Chapter 72).
11. Polysporin ointment should be applied to the cauterized area for 36 to 48 hr after the procedure.

COMPLICATIONS

1. Septal perforation from aggressive cautery
2. Caustic injury to the airway
3. Skin discoloration
4. Secondary bacterial infection of cautery site

References

Abelson TI, Witt WJ. Otolaryngologic procedures. In Roberts JR, Hedges JR (eds). *Clinical Procedures in Emergency Medicine* (2nd ed). Philadelphia, WB Saunders, 1991.
Ruddy RM (ed). Illustrated techniques of pediatric emergency procedures. In Fleisher GR, Ludwig S (eds). *Textbook of Pediatric Emergency Medicine* (3rd ed). Baltimore, Williams & Wilkins, 1993.

CHAPTER 70

Jim R. Harley

NASAL FOREIGN BODY REMOVAL

INDICATIONS

1. Presence of intranasal foreign body

CONTRAINDICATIONS

1. Agitated or highly uncooperative patient (these children require the use of sedation and analgesia)

EQUIPMENT

1. Topical anesthetic/vasoconstrictor (2 to 4% lidocaine mixed 50:50 with 0.5% oxymetazoline)

NOTE: Placing a tiny drop of peppermint oil into a 5- to 10-ml mixture of lidocaine and oxymetazoline will make the somewhat bitter taste and smell of that mixture much more tolerable for children.

2. Light source, preferably a head lamp
3. Nasal speculum (use the largest speculum that fits)
4. Foreign body removal device: bayonet forceps, alligator forceps, suction-tipped catheter, Fogarty catheter, cerumen ear loop, right-angle pick
5. Gloves

PROCEDURE

1. Unless the foreign body is quite anterior in the nasal cavity and easily reached, it is essential that the patient cooperate with the procedure. This may warrant the use of sedation and analgesia.
2. Spray or instill topical anesthetic/vasoconstrictor.
3. Using a good light source (and perhaps the nasal speculum), identify the size, shape, type, and location of the foreign body (Fig. 70-1*A*). These features will help to determine which removal device and technique is best suited.
4. The bayonet forceps or alligator forceps are best used for narrow foreign bodies or those with a small leading edge (Fig. 70-1*B*).

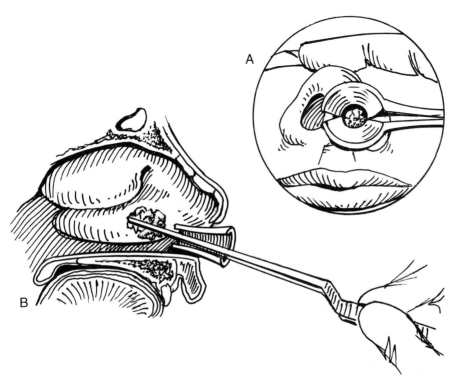

Figure 70–1. *A*, Using a nasal speculum and good light source, the presence and type of foreign body is identified. *B*, Cross-sectional view of foreign body removal using bayonet forceps and speculum.

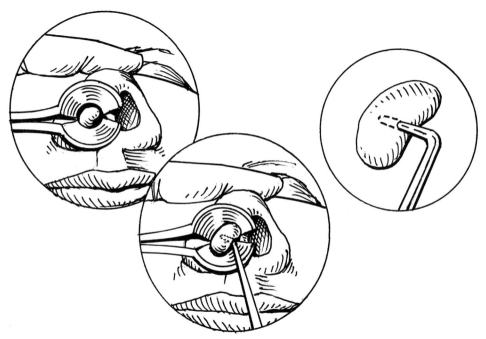

Figure 70–2. Removal of certain foreign bodies such as beans or beads may be facilitated by using a right-angle pick.

5. A suction-tipped instrument may be best suited for round, smooth-surfaced objects. If this fails, an angled ear loop can sometimes be placed behind the foreign body, scooping it out.
6. A right-angled pick may be best used for certain organic materials (e.g., beans) (Fig. 70–2).
7. A small Fogarty catheter (4 Fr) can be used to remove larger objects by passing the catheter behind the object, inflating the balloon, and removing the object.

COMPLICATIONS

1. Epistaxis
2. Aspiration of foreign body

References

Abelson TI, Witt WJ. Otolaryngologic procedures. In Roberts JR, Hedges JR (eds). *Clinical Procedures in Emergency Medicine* (2nd ed). Philadelphia, WB Saunders, 1991.
Ruddy RM (ed). Illustrated techniques of pediatric emergency procedures. In Fleisher GR, Ludwig S (eds). *Textbook of Pediatric Emergency Medicine* (3rd ed). Baltimore, Williams & Wilkins, 1993.

CHAPTER 71

Steven Krug

NASAL SEPTUM HEMATOMA EVACUATION

INDICATIONS

1. Presence of septal hematoma

CONTRAINDICATIONS

1. Bilateral septal hematomas (these should receive urgent evaluation by an otolaryngologist)

EQUIPMENT

1. Topical anesthetic/vasoconstrictor (2–4% lidocaine mixed 50:50 with 0.5% oxymetazoline)

NOTE: Placing a tiny drop of peppermint oil into the 5- to 10-ml mixture of lidocaine and oxymetazoline will make the somewhat bitter taste and smell of that mixture much more tolerable for children.

2. Hand-held atomizer or medicine dropper
3. Light source, preferably head lamp
4. Nasal speculum (the largest size that fits)
5. Scalpel, #11 blade
6. Cotton-tipped applicators
7. Cup forceps or iris scissors
8. Bayonet forceps
9. Packing material for anterior nasal pack (see Chapter 72)
10. Gloves

PROCEDURE

1. Spray or instill topical anesthetic/vasoconstrictor. Consider the use of sedation and analgesia. (See Chapter 3.)
2. Perform a careful examination of both sides of the septum, using a nasal speculum and a good light source (Fig. 71–1*A*).

NOTE: A septal hematoma should be considered in all patients with trauma to the nose or midface. An acute hematoma may not be ecchymotic; therefore, it may only

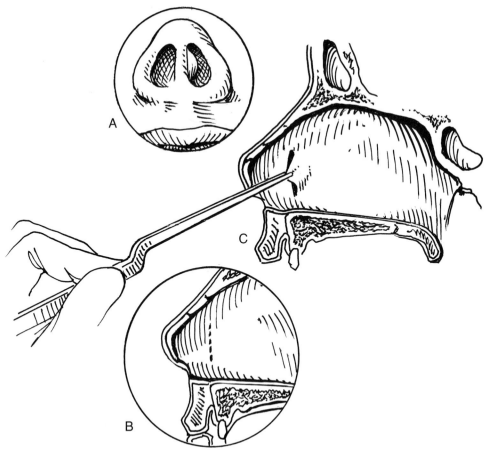

Figure 71–1. Evacuation of nasal septum hematoma: *A*, Appearance of hematoma at nares. *B*, Vertical incision through mucosa overlying hematoma. *C*, Blunt dissection of mucosa overlying hematoma.

be appreciated via palpation of the septum and notation of a boggy, fluctuant, or painful septum.

3. Make a long vertical incision through the nasal mucosa that overlies the hematoma (Fig. 71–1*B*).
4. Evacuate all blood or blot clot from the hematoma.
5. Using a pair of cup forceps or iris scissors, remove a small area of the incised mucosal surface (Fig. 71–1*C*). This will allow for continued drainage.
6. Insert an anterior nasal pack (see Chapter 72).
7. Place the patient on broad-spectrum antibiotic therapy.

COMPLICATIONS

1. Complications of untreated septal hematoma include the following: superinfection, abscess formation, destruction of septal cartilage, cavernous sinus thrombosis, meningitis

References

Abelson TI, Witt WJ. Otolaryngologic procedures. In Roberts JR, Hedges JR (eds). *Clinical Procedures in Emergency Medicine* (2nd ed). Philadelphia, WB Saunders, 1991.
Ruddy RM (ed). Illustrated techniques of pediatric emergency procedures. In Fleisher GR, Ludwig S (eds). *Textbook of Pediatric Emergency Medicine* (3rd ed). Baltimore, Williams & Wilkins, 1993.

CHAPTER 72

Steven Krug

NASAL PACKING

INDICATIONS

1. Recurrent epistaxis in spite of cautery attempts
2. Failure to obtain hemostasis (and inability to perform cautery) with application of topical anesthetic/vasoconstrictor

CONTRAINDICATIONS

None

EQUIPMENT

Anterior Pack

1. Topical anesthetic/vasoconstrictor (2 to 4% lidocaine mixed 50:50 with 0.5% oxymetazoline; or 4% cocaine solution)

NOTE: Placing a tiny drop of peppermint oil into 5- to 10-mL of the above solution will make the somewhat bitter taste and smell of that mixture much more tolerable for children.

NOTE: Cocaine is the single most potent topical vasoconstrictor and one of the most effective topical anesthetics available. It must be used with great caution when applied to mucous membranes.

2. Hand-held atomizer or medicine dropper
3. Light source, preferably head lamp
4. Nasal speculum (the largest size that fits)
5. Suction device
6. Gloves
7. Bayonet forceps
8. Vaseline gauze, ½ in
9. Gelfoam

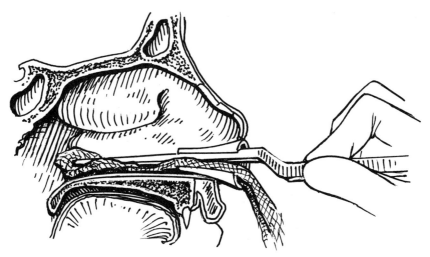

Figure 72–1. Anterior nasal packing using Vaseline gauze. First insert gauze along the floor of the nasal cavity with bayonet forceps.

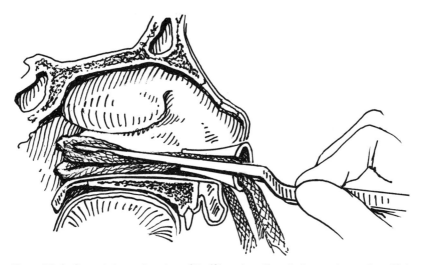

Figure 72–2. Gauze is layered on top of itself by reinsertion via the nasal speculum. Note "tail" dangling from nose.

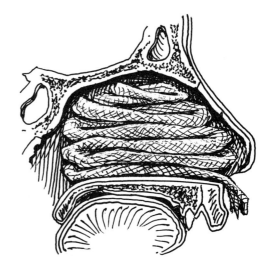

Figure 72–3. When procedure is complete, entire nasal cavity is tightly packed with gauze.

Posterior Pack

1-8. Same equipment as above.
9. Foley catheter, 10-14 Fr
10. 20-ml syringe
11. Saline
12. 2-in piece of ½-in suction tubing
13. Hoffmann clamp or hemostat

PROCEDURES

Anterior Packing

Gelfoam Method

1. Spray or instill topical anesthetic/vasoconstrictor drops.
2. Obtain good visualization of the nasal cavity with a nasal speculum and head lamp to determine the source (anterior versus posterior) of the bleeding. Have suction available.
3. Soak a folded piece of Gelfoam large enough to cover the area of bleeding in 4% cocaine solution or lidocaine-oxymetazoline.
4. Using a nasal speculum and bayonet forceps, apply the Gelfoam to the area of bleeding.
5. Apply direct pressure to the Gelfoam on the septum for 10 to 15 min.
6. The Gelfoam will expand to fill the anterior nasal chamber. It should remain in place for two or more days and will spontaneously adsorb and be expelled.

NOTE: Avitene is another self-adsorbing packing that can be applied to the nasal septum in a similar manner. It also has excellent hemostatic properties. It is, however, extremely expensive and should be reserved for special situations.

7. Insertion of a Merocel nasal tampon is a good commercial alternative to the use of Gelfoam or the insertion of a traditional gauze pack.

Gauze Method

1. Spray or instill topical anesthetic/vasoconstrictor drops. Consider the use of sedation and analgesia.
2. Obtain good visualization of the nasal cavity with a nasal speculum and head lamp to determine the source (anterior versus posterior) of the bleeding. Have suction available.
3. Using Vaseline-impregnated gauze, insert a length of gauze with a bayonet forceps along the floor of the nasal cavity. Leave a 2- to 3-cm "tail" hanging from the naris (Fig. 72-1).
4. Regrasp the "long-end" of the gauze dangling from the nose and reinsert it into the naris, above the gauze that has already been placed. The existing layer of gauze can be held in place by removing the speculum and reinserting the speculum over the existing gauze before inserting the next layer (Fig. 72-2).

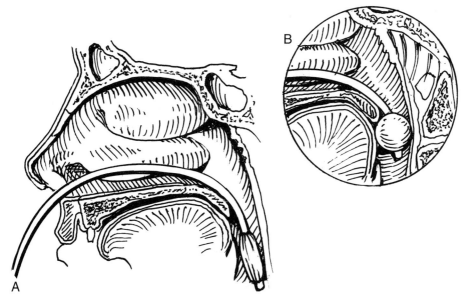

Figure 72–4. *A,* Posterior packing method requires insertion of a Foley catheter into the nasopharynx, to tamponade posterior bleeding source. *B,* Once the balloon is inflated, the Foley catheter should be pulled back, wedging it in place.

5. This procedure is completed until the nasal cavity has been filled (Fig. 72-3).
6. The patient should be placed on broad-spectrum antibiotic therapy.

NOTE: A nasal pack should not be left in place for more than 2 to 3 days.

Posterior Packing

NOTE: Posterior epistaxis is an uncommon but serious event in pediatric care. Suspicion of the presence of posterior bleeding should prompt immediate on-site

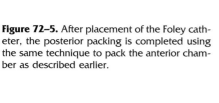

Figure 72–5. After placement of the Foley catheter, the posterior packing is completed using the same technique to pack the anterior chamber as described earlier.

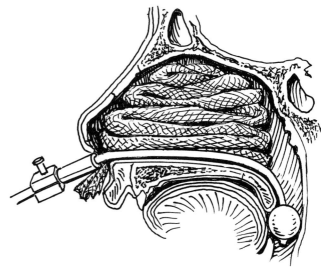

otolaryngology consultation. The method described here is not intended as definitive care but rather as a temporary "fix" until an otolaryngologist can evaluate the patient.

1. Spray or instill topical anesthetic/vasoconstrictor drops. Consider using sedation and analgesia.
2. Obtain good visualization of the nasal cavity with a nasal speculum and head lamp to determine the source (anterior versus posterior) of the bleeding. Have suction available.
3. Prepare a Foley catheter for insertion into the nasal cavity:
    a. Cut a 2-in length of ½-in suction tubing and slide this plastic sleeve over the entire length of the Foley catheter.
    b. Cut off the section of the Foley catheter distal to the balloon.
    c. Test the balloon by injecting 10 to 15 ml of saline; then deflate.
4. Insert the Foley catheter into the naris so that the balloon portion passes into the pharynx.
5. Reinflate the balloon with 10 to 15 ml of saline. Pull the Foley catheter back until the balloon is firmly wedged (Fig. 72-4).
6. Proceed with the application of an anterior pack around the catheter using Vaseline gauze and the technique described earlier.
7. Slide the plastic sleeve up until it wedges against the anterior pack.
8. Clamp the Foley catheter just distal to the plastic sleeve with a Hoffmann clamp or hemostat, securing it in place (Fig. 72-5).

COMPLICATIONS

1. Septal ulceration, pressure necrosis, perforation
2. Nasal alar necrosis
3. Bacterial rhinosinusitis
4. Toxic shock syndrome
5. Partial airway obstruction (hypercapnia and hypoxia)
6. Aspiration of packing material

References

Abelson TI, Witt WJ. Otolaryngologic procedures. In Roberts JR, Hedges JR (eds). *Clinical Procedures in Emergency Medicine* (2nd ed). Philadelphia, WB Saunders, 1991.
Ruddy RM (ed). Illustrated techniques of pediatric emergency procedures. In Fleisher GR, Ludwig S (eds). *Textbook of Pediatric Emergency Medicine* (3rd ed). Baltimore, Williams & Wilkins, 1993.

GASTROINTESTINAL AND URINARY TRACT PROCEDURES

CHAPTER 73

Michele Walsh-Sukys

INSERTION OF NASOGASTRIC TUBE

INDICATIONS

1. Decompression of stomach filled with air
2. Removal of gastric contents to prevent aspiration in a patient with an ileus or in a patient with an altered mental status

NOTE: A large-bore gastric tube may be indicated for the purpose of gastric detoxification, particularly if one hopes to remove pill fragments. This may require the passage of an orogastric rather than a nasogastric tube.

3. Removal of gastric contents for diagnostic purposes (e.g., blood)
4. Removal of an ingested substance to prevent toxicity
5. For instillation of activated charcoal to treat poisonings
6. To provide a route for enteral feedings when these cannot be taken orally

CONTRAINDICATIONS

1. Presence of a cribriform plate defect (relative—orogastric tube preferred)
2. Recent esophageal repair or perforation

EQUIPMENT

1. Gloves
2. Lubricant: sterile water, saline, or petroleum jelly
3. Nasogastric tube in size appropriate for patient (see Appendix A)

PROCEDURE

1. Estimate the depth of insertion by measuring the distance from the tip of the nose to the ear, and the ear to the subxiphoid notch.
2. Select an appropriate-sized nasogastric (NG) tube (one that is smaller than the nostril).
3. Lubricate the first several centimeters of the tube.
4. Gently insert the tube into the patient's nose with the tip oriented toward the nasal septum and the occiput (Fig. 73-1).
5. In patients who are old enough and able to cooperate, it may be helpful to have the patient in a sitting postion and swallowing sips of water while the NG tube is advanced.

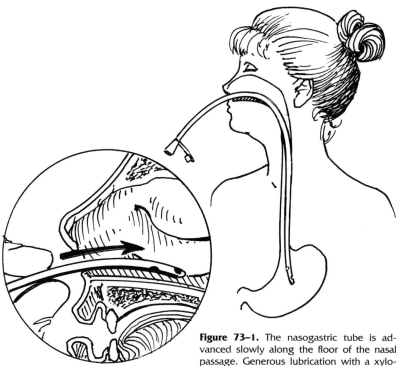

Figure 73–1. The nasogastric tube is advanced slowly along the floor of the nasal passage. Generous lubrication with a xylocaine-containing lubricant will facilitate placement and minimize patient discomfort. Preanesthetizing the naris with xylocaine is also recommended.

6. Gradually advance the tube to the measured depth.
7. Confirm gastric placement by injecting air into the tube while auscultating over the gastric bubble. If the tube is properly positioned, loud bubbling will be heard.
8. Place the tube to gravity drainage or to low (20 cm water) intermittent suction.
9. If the tube has an air channel as a component (frequently colored blue), avoid injecting any air or water into this port. This port is designed to prevent the tube from adhering to the gastric mucosa.
10. The gastric tube may also be inserted orally. This is less desirable, however, as it stimulates the gag reflex and is quite uncomfortable for the patient.

COMPLICATIONS

1. Emesis leading to aspiration
2. Intracranial placement in a patient with mid-facial injury and cribriform plate defect
3. Apnea or bradycardia in neonates
4. Hypoxia
5. Irritation and erosion of nasal mucosa with long-term placement
6. Insertion into the trachea or major bronchi. Malposition can usually be detected by the occurrence of frequent coughing and by the absence of bubbling over the stomach on the placement position check
7. Laceration or perforation of the posterior pharynx, esophagus, stomach, or duodenum (possibly avoided by using a lubricant and by using the softest tube available)
8. Placement of the tip in the duodenum (this malposition can usually be detected when large amounts of bile are returned from the tube that have an alkaline pH when tested)

CHAPTER 74

Steven Krug

GASTROSTOMY TUBE REPLACEMENT

INDICATIONS

1. Replacement of a dislodged, cracked, or obstructed gastrostomy tube

CONTRAINDICATIONS

1. Separation of the stomach from the abdominal wall
2. Significant bleeding from the stoma site

EQUIPMENT

1. Appropriate-sized replacement gastrostomy tube. In an emergency, a Foley catheter can be used as a short-term solution if a gastrostomy tube is not available.
2. Stylet (a rigid endotracheal tube stylet may be used for this purpose)
3. Sterile lubricant
4. Sterile saline
5. Gloves

PROCEDURE

1. Assess the patient to ensure the absence of bowel obstruction and examine the stoma site for bleeding. While bleeding may be due to local irritation, it can also be symptomatic of separation of the stomach from the abdominal wall. If the original tube is still present within the stoma, remove it by applying gentle but firm traction on the tube. If the patient has a tube with an inflatable cuff, remember to deflate the cuff first.
2. Identify the size and type of gastrostomy device. Pass a rigid stylet within the lumen of the new tube. Ensure that the stylet can easily be removed from the lumen in order to prevent accidental removal of the tube after insertion.

NOTE: A number of devices or instruments can be creatively employed as stylets.

3. For tubes with a mushroom-type head, advance the stylet and stretch the tube. This will straighten out the mushroom head (Fig. 74–1). For tubes with an inflatable cuff, test the patency of the cuff and then deflate.

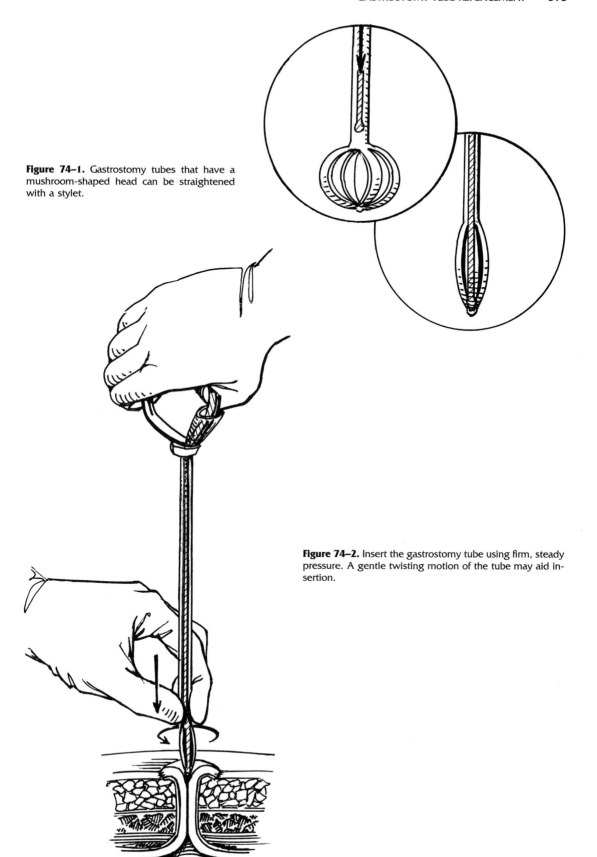

Figure 74–1. Gastrostomy tubes that have a mushroom-shaped head can be straightened with a stylet.

Figure 74–2. Insert the gastrostomy tube using firm, steady pressure. A gentle twisting motion of the tube may aid insertion.

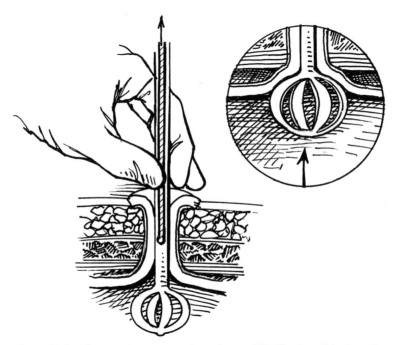

Figure 74–3. After insertion, remove the stylet carefully. Gently pull back on the tube until the resistance of the mushroom head against the inner surface of the stoma is felt.

4. Apply a generous amount of sterile lubricant to the tip of the tube.
5. With the child in a supine position, place the tip of the tube into the stoma. The nondominant hand should be used to guide the tube into the stoma with the heel of that hand placed directly on the abdominal wall. This will prevent slipping of the tube and will serve as a counterforce to steady, firm pressure applied by the dominant hand at the other end of the tube (Fig. 74–2).
6. The applied pressure should be perpendicular to the abdominal wall. It typically requires 15 to 45 sec of continued steady pressure to stretch the stoma adequately to accept the tube. It may take longer for tubes that have been dislodged.
7. As the stomach is entered, resistance will lessen dramatically. Care should be taken not to over-advance the tube. The tube should be advanced so that the entire mushroom tip (or the cuff) is well within the stomach.
8. Remove the stylet carefully so as not to pull the tube out. Once the stylet is removed, pull back on the tube gently. One should appreciate the resistance of the mushroom head on the inner surface of the stoma (Fig. 74–3). For cuffed tubes, inflate the cuff to its recommended volume and then pull back.
9. Determine the correct position of the tube using any or all of the following methods:
   a. Easy drainage of stomach contents noted from tube
   b. Easy infusion of sterile saline into the tube
   c. Infusion of air into the tube and plain radiograph findings of an air-filled stomach (and conversely, no free intra-abdominal air)
   d. Infusion of contrast dye into the stomach via the tube as documented on x-ray examination

COMPLICATIONS

1. Trauma to the stoma site with bleeding
2. Insertion of tube into the peritoneal space
3. Peritonitis, typically due to an intraperitoneal tube
4. Dislodging of the stomach from the abdominal wall
5. Gastric outlet obstruction

References

Ruddy RM (ed). Illustrated techniques of pediatric emergency procedures. In Fleisher GR, Ludwig S (eds). *Textbook of Pediatric Emergency Medicine* (3rd ed). Baltimore, Williams & Wilkins, 1993.
Samuels, L. Feeding tubes: Removal, replacement, and unclogging. In Roberts JR, Hedges JR (eds). *Clinical Procedures in Emergency Medicine* (2nd ed). Philadelphia, WB Saunders, 1991.

CHAPTER 75

Steven Krug

REDUCTION OF RECTAL PROLAPSE

INDICATIONS

1. Rectal prolapse with significant bleeding
2. Failure of spontaneous reduction for rectal prolapse

CONTRAINDICATIONS

1. Significant ischemia or gangrene of the prolapsed segment

EQUIPMENT

1. Gloves
2. Lubricant
3. 4 × 4 gauze

PROCEDURE

1. Place the child in a prone position as this will allow for greater visualization and access. The knee-chest prone position is ideal for the cooperative patient. In the anxious or uncooperative patient, consider the administration of sedation and analgesia. (See Chapter 3.)
2. Don gloves and lubricate gloves (or the prolapsed rectum).
3. Place two fingers from each hand on either side of the prolapsed tissue and slowly reduce the prolapse by placing alternating pressure on either side (Fig. 75-1). Placing a 4 × 4 gauze over the prolapse before attempting reduction may make the tissue less slippery.
4. Alternately, a gloved finger wrapped in gauze may be inserted into the rectal lumen with gentle pressure applied opposite to the direction of the prolapse.

COMPLICATIONS

1. Bleeding
2. Mucosal ulceration

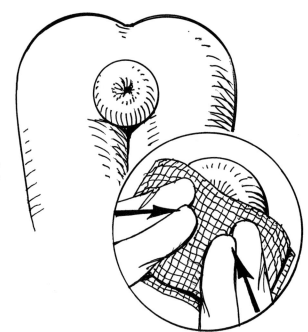

Figure 75–1. To reduce a rectal prolapse place two fingers on either side of the rectum. Alternate pressure on either side of the rectum.

References

Glauser JM. Rectal prolapse. In Roberts JR, Hedges JR (eds). *Clinical Procedures in Emergency Medicine* (2nd ed). Philadelphia, WB Saunders, 1991.

Ruddy RM (ed). Illustrated techniques of pediatric emergency procedures. In Fleisher GR, Ludwig S (eds). *Textbook of Pediatric Emergency Medicine* (3rd ed). Baltimore, Williams & Wilkins, 1993.

CHAPTER 76

Steven Krug

REDUCTION OF INGUINAL HERNIA

INDICATIONS

1. Reduction of herniated and/or incarcerated bowel to prevent strangulation ischemia

CONTRAINDICATIONS

1. Suspected ischemia or gangrene of the incarcerated bowel
2. Hydrocele

EQUIPMENT

1. Gloves

PROCEDURE

1. The patient should be placed in a supine position. A mild Trendelenburg position will also serve to reduce edema formation in the incarcerated bowel.
2. Steady pressure should be applied to the bowel within the inguinal canal to first reduce the contents of the incarcerated bowel back into the abdomen. This can be best achieved using both hands and placing uniform pressure on the entire length of bowel in the canal (Fig. 76-1). A pressure differential with slightly greater pressure at the distal aspect of the bowel will encourage the flow of bowel contents in the desired direction. Pressure may be required for up to 5 min.
3. Once the contents of the incarcerated bowel have been reduced, it is usually not difficult to reduce the bowel itself, unless a great amount of edema has formed.
4. If the reduction effort was unsuccessful, this is likely due to the associated patient discomfort and tensing of the abdomen. This may be defeated by using sedation and analgesia.

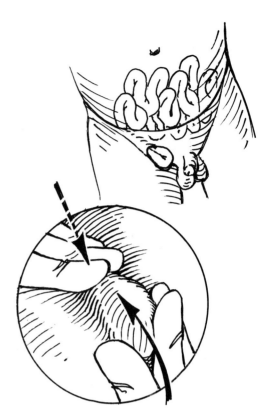

Figure 76–1. An inguinal hernia is reduced by applying uniform pressure to the bowel within the canal. Pressure may be required for up to 5 minutes before reduction occurs.

COMPLICATIONS

1. Injury to bowel from excessive compression
2. Perforation of bowel due to excessive compression- and/or incarceration-associated ischemia

References

Glauser JM. Abdominal hernia reduction. In Roberts JR, Hedges JR (eds). *Clinical Procedures in Emergency Medicine* (2nd ed). Philadelphia, WB Saunders, 1991.
Ruddy RM (ed). Illustrated techniques of pediatric emergency procedures. In Fleisher GR, Ludwig S (eds). *Textbook of Pediatric Emergency Medicine* (3rd ed). Baltimore, Williams & Wilkins, 1993.

CHAPTER *77*

Michele Walsh-Sukys

BLADDER CATHETERIZATION

INDICATIONS

1. To obtain urine for culture
2. To drain the bladder when spontaneous voiding is ineffective in emptying the bladder

CONTRAINDICATIONS

1. Genitourinary abnormalities
2. Extremely small infants (<750 g): size may be a relative contraindication as there may not be a catheter small enough to allow placement

EQUIPMENT

1. Sterile gloves
2. Drapes
3. Betadine
4. Catheter appropriate to the size of the patient (see Appendix A)
5. Two sterile cotton-tipped applicators
6. Sterile nonbactericidal lubricating ointment
7. 5- to 10-ml syringe

PROCEDURES

Female Catheterization

1. Prepare the urethra with Betadine in circular motions. Allow Betadine to dry.
2. Ask an assistant to retract the labia with the cotton-tipped applicators.
3. Apply the lubricating agent to the catheter tip.
4. Gently insert the catheter into the urethra, located between the clitoris and the vaginal introitus (Fig. 77-1A). If the catheter is inserted 4 to 5 cm and meets

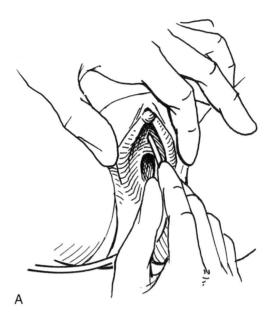

A

Figure 77–1. Bladder catheterization of a female (A) and a male patient (B). Urethral catheterization of the female is more challenging than catheterization of the male.

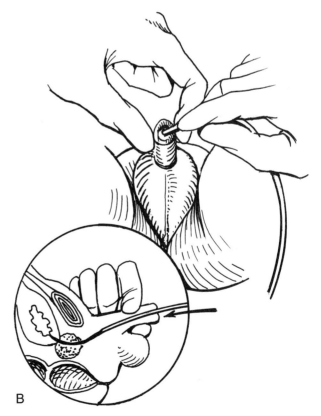

B

CHAPTER 78

John T. Kanegaye

PENILE ZIPPER ENTRAPMENT

INDICATIONS

1. Liberation of penile skin (usually foreskin) enmeshed in zipper

CONTRAINDICATIONS

Mineral Oil Technique

None

Wire Cutter Technique

1. Patient anxiety or agitation (relative risk of further injury during removal). Consider the use of sedation and analgesia. (See Chapter 3.)

EQUIPMENT

Mineral Oil Technique

1. Mineral oil
2. Supplies for local anesthetic infiltration (optional)

Wire Cutter Technique

1. Wire cutter appropriate to size and location of entrapment
2. Supplies for local anesthetic infiltration (optional)

PROCEDURES

Mineral Oil Technique

1. Apply mineral oil liberally to the zipper and to the entrapped skinfold.
2. In most cases, minimal traction will suffice to free the entrapped skin.
3. Local infiltration of lidocaine may be required in refractory cases.

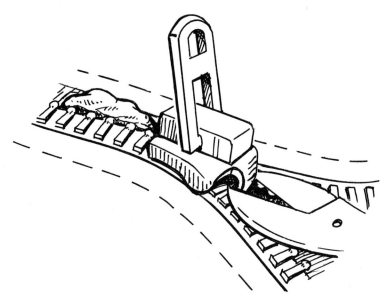

Figure 78–1. Divide the median bar of the zipper with wire cutters and separate the halves of the zipper.

Wire Cutter Technique

1. (Optional) Deliver subcutaneous wheal of local anesthetic.
2. Divide median bar of sliding portion of zipper with clippers and separate halves (Fig. 78-1)
3. Separate skin and zipper teeth.

COMPLICATIONS

1. Minor abrasions, skin maceration, hematoma, or bleeding may occur as a result of duration and severity of entrapment or from removal attempts or anesthetic infiltration.
2. Failure due to severity of entrapment. In such cases, more aggressive approaches may be necessary, including parenteral sedation and analgesia, local nerve blocks, and surgical/urologic consultation.

References

Kanegaye JT, Schonfeld N. Penile zipper entrapment: A simple and less threatening approach using mineral oil. Pediatr Emerg Care 9:90-91, 1993.
Snyder HM. Urologic emergencies. In Fleisher GR, Ludwig S, Henretig FM, et al (eds). *Textbook of Pediatric Emergency Medicine* (3rd ed). Baltimore, Williams & Wilkins, 1993, pp 1387-1395.

CHAPTER 79

John T. Kanegaye

REDUCTION OF PARAPHIMOSIS

INDICATIONS

1. Entrapment of foreskin proximal to glans

CONTRAINDICATIONS

1. Although the reduction of a true paraphimosis has no reasonable contraindications, the maneuver should be avoided in conditions that mimic paraphimosis (typically severe edema due to allergy, local irritation, or insect bite).

PROCEDURE

1. Restrain patient if necessary. Consider the use of sedation and analgesia. (See Chapter 3.)
2. (Optional) Deliver a dorsal or ring nerve block at the base of the penis.
   a. The dorsal nerve runs in a superficial position under the dorsal surface of the penis at a 12 o'clock position.
   b. Injection of 0.5 to 1.0 ml of 1% lidocaine (without epinephrine) just under the skin surface at the base of the penis should serve to block the nerve
   c. The patient may also require a subcutaneous ring block of the penis for complete analgesia. This can be accomplished with subcutaneous injection of 1% lidocaine in a circumferential fashion around the base of the penis.
3. (Optional) Reduce edema by squeezing the foreskin in various quadrants between the thumb and forefinger. Alternately, ice may be applied to the paraphimosis. Using a rubber glove partially filled with water and crushed ice and tied at the base, the penis is cooled by invaginating one of the glove's fingers into the ice water mixture.
4. Position thumbs over distal glans on both sides of meatus with fingers (index, long, and ring) placed behind the entrapped and edematous foreskin.
5. Push glans toward patient while exerting traction on foreskin, pulling it away from the patient and over the glans (Fig. 79-1).

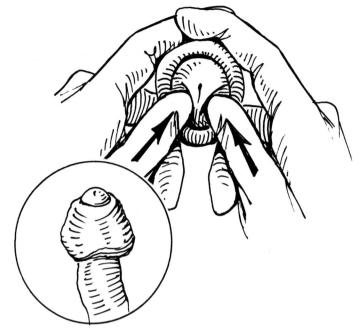

Figure 79–1. To reduce a paraphimosis, position thumbs over the distal glans. Push the glans toward the patient while exerting traction on the edematous foreskin. Pull the foreskin away from the patient and over the glans.

SUPPLEMENTAL TECHNIQUES

Percutaneous Reduction of Edema

Equipment

1. Antiseptic solution
2. 23-gauge or smaller needle

Procedure

1. Apply antiseptic to the foreskin.
2. Create one or two shallow puncture wounds in the foreskin.
3. Compress the foreskin between thumb and forefinger to express edema fluid.
4. Proceed with reduction.

   COMMENT: Although this technique permits rapid reduction of swelling, the clinical advantage compared with compression without puncture is unclear.

Hyaluronidase Technique

Equipment

1. Antiseptic solution
2. Hyaluronidase (1500 U vial)
3. 1% lidocaine without epinephrine
4. 1- or 3-ml syringe with fine-gauge (25-gauge or smaller) needle

Procedure

1. Apply antiseptic to the foreskin.
2. Reconstitute hyaluronidase with 4 ml of 1% lidocaine without epinephrine and infiltrate 0.25- to 1-ml at four equidistant sites or quadrants around the edematous foreskin.
3. After 10 min with or without application of an ice-water compress, reduction may proceed, with greatly reduced edema.

COMPLICATIONS

1. Post reduction edema occurs in almost all patients and requires no specific treatment.
2. Laceration of foreskin caused by shearing forces of a difficult reduction.
3. Risk of infection or vascular injury if a skin puncture or infiltration technique is used.
4. The hyaluronidase technique involves the local and systemic reactions described for both hyaluronidase and lidocaine. Because hyaluronidase is prepared from mammalian testicular tissue, a theoretical risk of antibody production exists. However, testicular degeneration has been described only in association with repeated exposure.
5. Incomplete reduction of the entire foreskin may give the false appearance of successful reduction with subsequent recurrence of the paraphimosis.
6. Complete failure of reduction attempt. Surgical or urologic consultation is warranted at this point for consideration of dorsal slit procedure.
7. Paraphimosis itself is a possible complication of procedures such as urethral catheterization or misadventures of foreskin care.

References

Barone JG, Fleisher MH. Treatment of paraphimosis using the "puncture" technique. Pediatr Emerg Care 9:298–299, 1993.

Illingworth RS. The Normal Child: Some Problems of the Early Years and Their Treatment (9th ed). New York, Churchill Livingstone, 1987, p 114.

Snyder HM. Urologic emergencies. In Fleisher GR, Ludwig S (eds). *Textbook of Pediatric Emergency Medicine* (3rd ed). Baltimore, Williams & Wilkins, 1993, pp 1387–1395.

APPENDIX A

PEDIATRIC TUBE AND CATHETER SIZES

Michele Walsh-Sukys and Steven Krug

Age	Endotracheal Tube (I.D. mm)	Suction Catheter (Fr)	Gastric Tube (Fr)	Chest Tube (Fr)	Urinary Catheter (Fr)
Premie	2.5–3.0 uncuffed	5	5	8–10	3–5
Term infant	3.0–3.5 uncuffed	5–8	5–8	10–12	5–8
6 mo	3.5–4.0 uncuffed	8	8–10	14–20	8
1 yr	4.0–4.5 uncuffed	8–10	10	18–24	8–10
2 yr	4.5 uncuffed	10	10	16–24	10
4 yr	5.0 uncuffed	10–12	10–12	20–28	10–12
6 yr	5.5 uncuffed	10–12	12–14	24–32	10–12
8 yr	6.0 cuffed	12	14–18	28–32	12
10 yr	6.5 cuffed	12	18	32–40	12
Adolescent	7.0–8.0 cuffed	12–14	18	34–42	12

Alternative Methods for Rapid Size Determination:

1. Endotracheal Tube Size (I.D. mm) = (16 + Age) ÷ 4

2. Endotracheal Tube Depth of Insertion
     Oral: Newborns: 7–10 cm
              Older Children: Age + 10 cm
     Nasal: Older Children: Age + 13 to 15 cm

I.D. mm, internal diameter in millimeters; Fr, French.

APPENDIX **B**

RESUSCITATION DRUG DOSAGES

Sally Reynolds

Primary Life Support Drugs

Drug	Indications	Route/Dose	Precautions
Epinephrine	Asystole or pulseless arrest	*First dose:* IV/IO 0.01 mg/kg *or* 0.1 ml/kg (1:10,000) ET: 0.1 mg/kg *or* 0.1 ml/kg (1:1000) *Initial adult dose:* 1 mg; may escalate to 2–5 mg IV push every 3–5 min *Subsequent doses:* IV/IO/ET 0.1 mg/kg *or* 0.1 ml/kg (1:1000) IV/IO doses as high as 0.2 mg/kg (1:1000) may be effective Repeat every 3–5 min	1. Not to be mixed with bicarbonate or calcium salts 2. May cause tachycardia, ventricular ectopy
	Unstable bradycardia	IV/IO 0.01 mg/kg 0.1 ml/kg (1:10,000) ET: 0.1 mg/kg 0.1/ml/kg (1:1000)	
Atropine	1. Second line drug for symptomatic bradycardia unresponsive to airway management, ventilation, and epinephrine 2. Block reflex bradycardia during intubation	IV/IO/ET 0.02 mg/kg Minimum dose 0.1 mg or may have paradoxic bradycardia Maximum single dose in children 0.5 mg Maximum single dose in adolescent 1.0 mg May repeat every 5 min, to a maximum total dose of 1 mg in a child and 2 mg in an adolescent	1. Bradycardia often due to hypoxia 2. Adequate patient ventilation
Adenosine	Supraventricular tachycardia	*First dose:* IV/IO 0.05 to 0.1 mg/kg *Second dose:* IV/IO 0.1 to 0.2 mg/kg *Third dose:* IV/IO 0.3 mg/kg Maximum single dose 12 mg	1. Given as very rapid IV bolus 2. Half-life: < 10 sec

Drug	Indications	Route/Dose	Precautions
Bretylium	Use as second line drug for ventricular fibrillation or ventricular tachycardia	*First dose:* IV/IO 5 mg/kg *Second dose:* IV/IO 10 mg/kg Maximum total dose 30 mg/kg	1. Rapid IV bolus 2. May cause hypotension 3. Not to be used in digitalis-induced dysrhythmia
Calcium chloride	1. Given for documented hypocalcemia 2. Considered for hyperkalemia, hypermagnesemia, calcium channel blocker overdose	IV/IO 20 mg/kg *or* 0.2 ml/kg of 10% sol Maximum dose 500 mg	1. Given slowly 2. Not mixed with bicarbonate 3. May cause severe extravasation burns
Naloxone	1. Narcotic overdose 2. Unknown toxic ingestion	ET/IO/IM/IV 0.1 mg/kg up to 20 kg >20 kg: give 2 mg initially May be repeated within 2–5 min to a total of 10 mg	1. May cause withdrawal symptoms 2. Effective half-life 30–60 min
Sodium bicarbonate	1. Prolonged arrest 2. Documented metabolic acidosis	IV/IO Child: 1 mEq/kg 8.4% solution Neonate: 2 mEq/kg 4.2% solution	1. Adequate ventilation 2. Slow infusion
Glucose	Hypoglycemia	IV/IO Child: D_{25} 2–4 ml/kg Neonate: D_{10} 2 mL/kg	Dextrostick to be checked, as too much glucose may make patient hyperosmolar
Lidocaine	1. Ventricular fibrillation 2. Pulseless ventricular tachycardia	IV/IO/ET 1–1.5 mg/kg Maximum single dose: 100 mg May repeat dose every 5–10 min to maximum dose of 5 mg/kg	1. High plasma concentrations possibly producing myocardial and circulatory depression 2. May cause CNS depression and seizures

Drugs Used For Intubation

Drug	Indications	Route/Dose	Precautions
Atropine	1. Blockade of reflex bradycardia	IV/IO 0.02 mg/kg Minimum dose 0.1 mg	
Thiopental	1. Closed head injury 2. Intracranial hypertension	IV/IO 2–5 mg/kg Onset: 20–60 sec	1. Hypotensive or hypovolemic patients 2. Not for use in status asthmaticus
Midazolam	1. Sedation alternative to thiopental 2. Hypovolemic or hypotensive patient	IV/IO 0.1 mg/kg Up to maximum 5 mg	
Ketamine	1. Status asthmaticus	IV/IO 1–2 mg/kg	1. Not for use in head injury 2. May cause laryngospasm

Appendix continued on following page

Drugs Used for Intubation (*Continued*)

Drug	Indications	Route/Dose	Precautions
Succinylcholine	1. Neuromuscular blockade 2. Ideal onset and duration for rapid sequence induction	IV/IO 1–2 mg/kg Onset: 30–60 sec Duration: 3–12 min	1. In children >5 yr old defasciculating dose of pancuronium to be used prior to succinylcholine 2. Avoid use in presence of increased intracranial or intraoccular pressure 3. Avoid use in crush injuries or severe burns
Rocuronium	1. Neuromuscular blockade 2. Optional agent for head trauma	IV/IO 0.6–0.8 mg/kg Onset: 45–75 sec Duration: 25–75 min	1. Lengthy duration of paralysis
Vecuronium	1. Neuromuscular blockade 2. May be used in head trauma	IV/IO 0.2 mg/kg Onset: 90–120 sec Duration: 25–60 min	1. Lengthy duration of paralysis
Pancuronium	1. Neuromuscular blockade	IV/IO 0.1 mg/kg Onset: 2–3 min Duration: 25–60 min	1. Lengthy duration of paralysis
Lidocaine	1. Prevent ICP elevation in head trauma	IV/IO 1.0–1.5 mg/kg	1. Can cause cardiovascular depression

Vasoactive Drug Infusions

Drug	Add to D_5W to Make 100 ml	Infuse	Dose Delivers	Therapy Range
Dopamine	60 mg	1 ml/kg/hr	10 μg/kg/min	1–5 renal μg/kg/min 5–15 cardiac 10–20 vasopressor

Indications:
1. Hypotension or poor perfusion in a patient with good intravascular volume and a stable rhythm

Medication / Indications / Precautions				
Precautions: 1. Produces tachycardia; increases myocardial O_2 demand, arrhythmias, and hypertension 2. Doses higher than 20 µg/kg/hr can cause ischemia 3. Extravasation can cause tissue necrosis				2–20 µg/kg/min
Dobutamine — *Indications:* 1. Treatment of severe congestive heart failure or cardiogenic shock. *Precautions:* 1. Tachycardia and tachyarrhythmias 2. Extravasation may cause tissue necrosis	60 mg	1 ml/kg/hr	10 µg/kg/min	
Epinephrine — *Indications:* 1. Used to treat poor perfusion or hypotension in a patient with good intravascular volume and a stable rhythm 2. Also used for hemodynamically unstable bradycardia. *Precautions:* 1. Can produce significant supraventricular or ventricular tachycardias and ventricular ectopy 2. May produce profound vascular constriction that compromises extremity and skin profusion 3. Increases myocardial O_2 consumption which can lead to ischemia	0.6 mg	1 ml/kg/hr	0.1 µg/kg/min	0.1–1.0 µg/kg/min

Appendix continued on following page

Vasoactive Drug Infusions *(Continued)*

Drug	Add to D$_5$W to Make 100 ml	Infuse	Dose Delivers	Therapy Range
Isoproterenol	0.6 mg	1 ml/kg/hr	0.1 µg/kg/min	0.5–1.0 µg/kg/min
Indications: 1. Hemodynamically unstable bradycardia after atropine has failed 2. Torsades de pointes *Precautions:* 1. May decrease coronary perfusion, decrease diastolic blood pressure, and increases mycardial O$_2$ demand 2. DO NOT USE to treat cardiac arrest.				
Lidocaine	120 mg	1 ml/kg/hr	20 µg/kg/min	20–50 µg/kg/min
Indications: 1. Recurrent ventricular tachycardia, ventricular fibrillation and ventricular ectopy *Precautions:* 1. Do not use in bradycardia with wide complex escape beats 2. May cause myocardial depression, disorientation, seizures 3. Decrease dose in patients with hepatic insufficiency				

IV = intravenous
IO = intraosseous
ET = endotracheal

INDEX

Note: Page numbers in *italics* refer to illustrations; page numbers followed by t refer to tables.

ISBN 0-7216-3789-2

90038

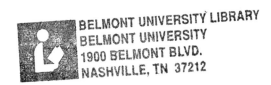